COMMON ANIMAL DISEASES

COMMON ANIMAL DISEASES

Dr. S.K. Singh

Oxford Book Company
Jaipur ▪ New Delhi

Published By

Oxford Book Company

Regd. Off. "Bony Residency", Gate No. 2
Opp. Tilak Public School, Vishweswariya Nagar,
Gopalpura Road, Jaipur - 302018, India
Ph: 0141 - 2761280, Telefax: 2761381
email - oxfordbookjpr@gmail.com
website - oxfordbookcompany.com

Delhi Office: 102, 1st Floor, Satyam House,
4327/3, Ansari Road, Darya Ganj,
New Delhi - 110002, India
Ph: 011-45652440

Distributed By

KEYA INTERNATIONAL PRESS LLP
E-mail: keyainternationalpressllp@gmail.com

Published in India, 2025

ISBN : 9789391096571

Typeset by Shivangi Computers, Jaipur

Printed and bound in India by Thomson Press Ltd.,
New Delhi

Contents

Preface

Dairy cattle are susceptible to the same diseases as beef cattle. Many diseases and pests plague the cattle industries of the world, the more serious ones being prevalent in the humid and less developed countries. One of the more common diseases to be found in the developed countries is brucellosis, which has been controlled quite successfully through vaccination and testing. This disease produces undulant fever in humans through milk from infected cows. Leptospirosis, prevalent in warm-blooded animals and humans, is caused by a spirochete and results in fever, loss of weight, and abortion. Bovine tuberculosis has been largely eliminated; where it has not, it can infect other warm-blooded animals, including humans. Test and slaughter programs have proved effective. Rabies, caused by a specific virus that also can infect most warm-blooded animals, is usually transmitted through the bite of infected animals, either wild or domestic. Foot-and-mouth disease has been eliminated from most of North America, some Central American countries, Australia, and New Zealand.

The rest of the world is still plagued by the disease, which attacks all cloven-footed animals. Humans are mildly susceptible to this organism. Successful vaccinations have been developed for blackleg, malignant edema, infectious bovine rhinotracheitis (or red nose), and several other diseases. Anaplasmosis, common to most tropical and semitropical regions, is spread by the bite of mosquitoes and flies. Anthrax, caused by a generally fatal bacterial infection, has been largely eliminated in the United States and western Europe. Rinderpest, still common to Asia and Europe, is caused by a specific virus that produces high fever and diarrhea. An infectious fever sometimes called nagana, caused by the tsetse fly, attacks both cattle and horses and is prevalent in central and southern Africa, as well as in the Philippines. Grass tetany and milk fever both result from metabolic disturbances. Bloat, caused by rapid gas formation in the rumen, or first compartment of the stomach, is sometimes fatal unless relieved. Pinkeye is an infectious inflammation of the eyes spread by flies or dust and is most serious in cattle having white pigmentation around one or both eyes. Mastitis, an inflammation of the udder, is caused by rough handling or by infection. Vibriosis, a venereal disease that causes abortion; pneumonia, an inflammation of the lungs; and shipping fever all cause serious losses and are difficult to control except through good management. Broad-spectrum antibiotics (antibiotics that are effective against various microorganisms), as well as powerful and specific pharmaceuticals, are effective and profitable means of keeping cattle herds healthy. Vermifuges, which destroy or expel parasitic worms, and insecticides, which kill harmful insects, are also highly effective and much used.

An infectious blood disease caused by the rickesttsial parasites Anaplasma marginale and Anaplasma centrale. It occurs primarily in warm tropical climate areas. The disease is not contagious but it can be transmitted most commonly by ticks but also by using contaminated needles, dehorning equipment, castrating knives, tattoo instruments, biting flies and mosquitoes. This parasite destroys red blood cells. It causes anemia, fever, weight loss, breathlessness, uncoordinated movements, abortion and death. Diagnosis is based on clinical signs and the examination of blood under microscope for evidence of the parasite. A highly infectious and fatal disease of mammals and humans. It is caused by a relatively large spore-forming rectangular shaped bacterium called Bacillus anthracis. Most outbreaks occur in areas where animals have previous died of anthrax, as the spores remain viable for decades. The predominant sign in cattle with anthrax is a progression from a normal appearance to dead in a matter of hours. Most animals are simply found dead. Once an outbreak begins in the animals may be observed with signs of weakness, fever, excitement followed by depression, difficulty breathing, uncoordinated movements and convulsions. Bloody discharges from the natural body openings as well as edema in different parts of the body are sometimes observed. After death, the animal's body rapidly decomposes.

The present book has been carefully compiled and edited to meet the long felt needs of increasingly number of students and researchers who have to deal with the different aspects of animal diseases.

— Dr. S.K. Singh

Chapter 1

Common Diseases : Prevention and Treatment in Cattle

If poisonous trees or shrubs over hang the fence line animals can nibble at heir leaves.

Goats will easily lean against the trunk, or the garden fence to reach the leaves. Also: Animals have been poisoned when trimmings have been discarded over the garden fence.

Some plants remain poisonous even thought they are "old and dried". Make sure pet lambs, or kids don't have access to poisonous plants if kept in the garden area.

All parts of this tree are toxic. It contain a substance which can stops the heart beating!!!.

Often the animal is found dead. If your animal eats YEW.. There is really nothing that can be done other than calling the vet, and getting surgery done. ie open the rumen and remove all traces of YEW.

After eating Rhododendron the animal may remain ill for several days.

The animal may kick at its stomach. (kicking at the stomach is an indication of pain.)

It may vomit. (Perhaps the only reason that an animal may vomit)

It may have difficulty breathing. Usually the animal will survive.

All parts of this plant are poisonous. The pods and seeds are very toxic. Signs and symptoms include: Neurological symptoms, (excitement, convulsions, and this is followed by death.) YES: Eating laburnum is usually fatal. The vet may administer a sedative to minimise the nervous signsand this can allow the animal to expel the toxins from it's body.

All parts of the plant are poisonous. Animals have been poisoned by eating the seeds.

Signs and Symptoms: There may be some neurological signs and symptoms, flowed by a

Coma, then death. Hemlock has been blamed for birth defects in young animals.

Ragwort can cause irreversible changes in the liver. The animal (after eating it) may not show symptoms for some time, until suddenly changes appear. The abdomen becomes enlarges and swollen. The animal appears very dull. This is irreversible. These is no cure. The animal should be culled. Normally animals avoid ragwort. They don't like the taste.

If ragwort is in hay the animal may NOT recognise it's unpalatable taste, and eat it.

Animals may eat bracken when feed is scarce. The fresh plant is not particularly palatable to animals. It has been known to be caught up in hay, where the taste is more palatable. Bracken can cause scouring, with blood in the faeces. t can cause severe anaemia because of a thrombocytopenia. (a deficiency in thrombocytes essential for blood coagulation).

Well fed animals seldom "choose" to feed on trees.. Problems occur when animals eat cuttings, or bits of branch or leaves that have arrived in their feed.. by the wind, or tossed over the garden fence. Several trees are known to cause abortions, or premature births in late pregnancy.. Worse still cows often retain the placenta, which may lead to, endometritis (uterine infection) and a visit by the vet. Fence off the offending trees. But if living in a windy area, be aware that twigs, leaves and branches may be carried into the pasture by the wind. An outbreak of abortions in a dairy herd was attributed to bits of macrocarpa having being caught up in the hay when the hay was made.

Even in a "dead state" clearly macrocarpa leaves can still cause abortions/premature births. Ponderosa Pine: (Pinus ponderosa Laws (USA) Lodgepole pine, Monterey Cypress. Leyland Cypruss:-A cross between the monterey cypress and the Alaskan Cedar. It was a popular tree, and planted for shelter and it's rapid growth. It joins the list of trees that can cause abortions. Macrocarpa is a well known abortion ogenic in cattle, and possibly deer. There are many macrocarpa shelter belts in existence.

(NZ cattle DO need shelter from wind, and cold weather.) Pine tree needles: (I'm told) Have also been blamed for causing abortions in cattle. (I don't know what species of pine are responsible.)

New paint may cover the old lead paint. Ensure that animals cant have access to pealing paint. Worse: Ashes from timber with old lead based paint on it: There is a suggestion that a lead content will remain in the ashes.

Chemicals: Insecticides, herbicides, rat poison, slug bait, petrol. Cattle have been known to 'sample' these. This has mainly occured when cattle (in particular) have managed to get into a farm building.. The cattle were curious, and possibly hungry. Their tongues can flip open (some) hooks, and bolt catches. They can knock over a drum, thus spilling the contents over the floor. These can be fatal to children also. They need to be keep them under lock and key.

Bloat occurs because of the fertilizers used today".-(totally False).

Bloat has been occurring for centuries !!A book printed in 1850 has this to say about bloat: Hoven, or Bloating: – This often follows the feeding of large quantities of green fodder. Clover, and alpha (Lucerne) contribute to the problem.

Before Modern Farming Times: Any sign of cattle bloating the farmer would chase the animal to encourage it to burp. One elderly farmer I spoke to reckoned his cows would position themselves facing up hill so they could burp more easily. Actual numbers of deaths from bloat is always vague, because the rumen naturally bloats up after the animal has died

Ruminant digestion involves micro-organisms which are needed to digest fibrous feeds.

During digestion these micro-organisms produce large quantities of gas.

The gas needs to be burped/eructated, and so frequent burping is an essential part of the digestion. Cattle burping is usually unnoticeable, and yet it happens roughly once a minute, increasing to 3 or more times each minute at peak times. In bloat the distention of the rumen by gas, or other contents, interferes or halts the normal burping process.

It is at the non reproductive stage (before and after the pre flowering stage) that legumes in pasture are most likely to cause bloat. Alpha (or Lucerne) & clover are the common legumes) Some farmers blame lush grass also. Spring is the main time of year when bloat is a danger. BUT: Autumn also, when the weather: moisture, heat, cool evenings: Farmers have been taken completely by surprise with the sudden occurrence of bloat in their animals. *If you have a bloated animal, talk about it tell neighbouring farmers, so they can take precautions with their stock. There is a suggestion that some animals eat mainly the legumes in the pasture, rather than a mix of grass & legumes.

Ensure that on heat cows are protected from bloat. A cow actively on heat may eat very little. She may make up for this later by gorging great quantities of lush pasture.

The predisposition to bloat seems to be inherited so there is merit in not breeding from animals that bloat easily. If you cull any frequent "bloaters" You'll get cash rather than finding a corpse in your paddock. In a given paddock, a few animals in the herd will bloat, and the others won't. Feeding out hay prior to releasing animals into lush pasture has been used as a method to reduce bloat. If you're using small bales, some drench solution could be applied to the cut side of the bale. Putting hungry animals onto lush pasture should be avoided. Some opt to transfer their animals to a fresh paddock in the afternoon after their stock has had a "good feed" in the morning. Reducing the proportion of legumes isn't a good idea. Legumes are a valuable source of protein and some minerals.

There are many on the market, and these are available from your vet and farm supplies stores. There are various solutions available and different ways to have it available for your stock:-drench, trough treatment, block, capsules etc. If you drench your animals: This way you KNOW the animal has had sufficient solution. Other methods of giving cattle anti foaming agent are good. But you cannot be 100% sure they have received the treatment. Read and obey the instructions on the wrapping. (Usually bloat prevention is continued through spring until the legumes reach their flowering stage.)

Rumensin Users: It does give some bloat control, but it should NOT be relied upon to give 100% bloat prevention. Bloat: Can take farmers by surprise!!! Some farmers start their precautionary methods prior to severe bloat conditions, and others wait until they presume the conditions and pasture could cause bloat. Autumn is the season where farmers have been taken by surprise.. and in big commercial herds this has meant the loss of several animals. Tell neighbours, & other farmers if you've had bloat in your herd. (You would have appreciated being aware of the likelihood of bloat yourself.)

Usually the container of anti-bloat solution has instructions re drenching a moderately bloated animal. (if you have some solution.) Alternatives: Use the vegetable oil from you kitchen. (It must be a vegetable oil, and not a mineral oil) Administer about 200mls of a vegetable oil. Use a narrow necked bottle for administering, it will be easier to maneuver.

(Some farmers reckon they've had good results by giving beer for mild bloat.)

You can't miss severe bloating. !!! They're out like a huge balloon. The left side in particular is huge and it is rounded from her spine to her underneath. The Right side is extremely bulged out also. Tap this bulge, and it responds like a drum. The animal appears uncomfortable and it is gasping for breath. The tongue protrudes.

If you have your cell phone on you RING YOUR VET NOW. It may take too long for a vet to get to you while the animal is in this critical state. Get instructions from the vet, and stay in touch with the vet. (While you're phoning the vet you could be heading for the house to get a bloat knife, or even a sharp, preferably sharp ended knife.)

Carry all sorts of things with them in the container on their bikes/ quads:

> *(Notebook & pen, pliers, twine, and perhaps a *Trocar and cannula, or a bloat knife.)*
>
> *(The cannula is a metal sleeve that fits over the trocar (trocar: the spear part of the duo).. The hollow cannula stays in place in the animal while the trocar is removed. This allows gas and gunk to escape.) The alternative of not taking the next step will be DEATH from asphyxiation, and the heart will fail, and this is due to the huge pressure of the rumen against vital organs. If you do not have a trocar and cannula, or a bloat knife. Use a very sharp knife. (One with a sharp pointed end.) You're going to have to stab your animal. The sharp knife, (or assembled trocar and cannula together), need to be "plunged" into the animal.*

Left side, somewhere between the ribs and the pelvis (basically, where the swelling is the greatest.) (If using a knife, Place you're thumb over the blunt end so the knife doesn't slip and cut you. You'll need to make a cut also.) The response can be dramatic, with an explosion of escaping gas, and gunk. You may have to clear out some of the frothy gunk yourself by hand. Contact the vet again.. Anti foaming agents are often added to the rumen to reduce frothing. The vet will administer antibiotics, and suture up the animal.

It is less severe in sheep than in cattle. It is always wise to vaccinate against clostridial disease (5-in-1) before sheep go out onto lush spring pasture, because bloat may occur with pulpy kidney. There are anti bloat treatments for sheep. Sheep can be sat on their butts, to rub their stomachs. They can take some vegetable oil also.. This will encourage them to burp.

Mineral Deficiencies

The feed is very short, buying in feed is an option. Feeding meal to your stock is one option. (There may be cheaper options) Introducing meal or new feeds to the diet must be done *very gradually*. This is to allow the animals rumen to manufacture 'bugs' essential for the 'digestion' of this new feed. (Stock will need extra water because of the dryness of the feed.)

Warm weather is a contributing factor in this group of diseases. Arguably New Zealand's weather is changing, and the conditions listed below are appearing out of their usual geographical area... Cattle and sheep with liver fluke appear unthrifty, and often have oedema around the jaw line. The long life cycle of this parasite involves a tiny snail, plus a suitable warm, wet environment (e.g. around springs, bogs) for the fluke eggs to hatch.

Facial Eczema

Facial eczema can occur in cattle, sheep and goats. The disease is caused by toxins in the spores of a saprophytic fungus (Pithomyces chartum) which live in dead vegetative material in pastures (esp ryegrass). The *fungal growth is enhanced by humid, wet, warm weather*. This is when spore levels rise rapidly. Animal livers damaged by the toxin (sporidesmin) cannot properly metabolise phylloerythrin, and it accumulates in the peripheral blood. This leads to a photosensitisation reaction in nonpigmented skin. Infected animals become photophobic, and seek shade.

Non pigmented areas of the body (white areas) may become severely ulcerated, with the accompanying symptoms of, itching, scabs, swollen infected areas, plus loss of appetite. Signs and symptoms may not always be obvious... the animal may have subclinical facial eczema. In a post mortems facial eczema livers are smaller, with much fibrous tissue. Animals *affected* should have shade, cool water, and a good diet. Prevention: Feed high levels of zinc BEFORE stock are at risk. Zinc is not a treatment

Death from heat stress in NZ is fortunately rare. Many animals show some of the signs of stress in a very hot especially humid sunny days. Black animals are prone. Fat cattle are more prone than lean ones. Visible *symptoms include*: Cattle seeking shade. They will align themselves with the sun. They will breath with their mouths open. They may pant, and salivate.

Ruminant digestion heats their bodies..

SO your animals need COOL water to drink.

Give them a fresh paddock later on in the day when the temperatures are NOT SO HOT.

Heat stress can have longer lasting effects-

lowering their feed intake, their milk production. & breeding efficiency.-and even DEATH.-

Shelter really is a MUST HAVE.

Seriously Consider *planting trees* for shelter and shade. Trees improve the 'look' of your farm, and you gain the timber value. Deciduous trees, provide shade for stock, their shade minimises evaporation in pasture they shelter over summer. Yet leafless in winter their shade is minimal. The leaves in autumn contribute to the soils litter layer, thus adding to soil health.

Nursing a Sick Animal

Warmth: Rumen fermentation provides warmth for the animal. You can also provide warmth by covering a sick animal with a blanket or cover. Food: Have water, grass, hay, or and molasses on offer. Position: the animal in a sitting position aids 'belching'. The heavy weight of the animal can restrict circulation to its limbs. So position it in a natural sitting position. In a cow the weight bearing hind leg (the foot part) should only just be visible under the udder. Prop it up with a bale of hay if necessary. Transporting sick cattle: When faced with moving a sick animal that is unable to stand. Use either a sturdy gate, or a couple of sheets of overlapped lengthwise roofing iron secured to timber at the top and base.

The plan is to use a rope to attach it to the tractor, and to tow this makeshift stretcher. Roll the animal onto the stretcher. Make sure limbs dont collide with gateways. You may have to secure the animals head with a rope. The Hospital Paddock: It may be close to the house or shed for convenience. With a 'hospital paddock' near a major road, consider the view motorists will get...Animals stuck in mud: Secure a chain and hook, or a rope (dont use a slip knot) around the animals neck. Attach to the tractor. Gently pull the animal to safety.

Sometimes hoof problems are caused by injury e.g. sharp stones, nails, glass, barbed wire (perhaps hidden amongst growing grass). A small stone, or a stick may be lodged between the claws (just remove it). If there is an infection in the hoof, to treatment let any pus out. Consider getting Vet assistance if inexperienced with hooves. They can locate painful areas accurately, and with their experience they can differentiate between healthy and non healthy tissue.

Examining a Hoof: Immobilise the animal, in a crush, or a bail Use a rope handy to elevate, and immobilise the animals leg.

Learn from Your Vet: Ask them to explain what they are doing. Ask about preventing hoof problems. The Vet may administer an antibiotic.

Footrot

Cause: Bacterial-often spread by introducing an infected sheep into the flock. The bacteria causing footrot does not invade healthy hooves. Transmission of the disease usually occurs in wet conditions.

Preventing the Disease: Some farmers will send contaminated animals 'to the works'. A vaccination is available. Quarantine newly purchased sheep if concerned. Romneys are footrot resistant.

Wounds

Deep Wounds: These are best stitched by a vet when they are very fresh.

If a wound contains pus, the pus must be 'let out' for the wound to heal.

Cleaning a Small Contaminated Wound: Make up a solution 100mls of boiling water, with a teaspoon of salt dissolved in it. You'll need some cotton wool swabs. Wipe over the area once, then discard the swab, repeat with a clean swab until wound is much cleaner.

Clean Fresh Wounds: Spray the area with an iodine solution.

Clots in the milk, or a hard, swollen section of your animal's udder may be the clue that your animal has mastitis.

The udder may be sore when touched. She may be feeling unwell also.

Mastitis Means: Inflammation of the mammary gland.

Some mastitis causing bacteria can be picked up "from the environment": (dung, mud, soil, water, & flies.)

Transfer from cow to cow, is common, especially in machine milked animals.

It can also be transferred from one quarter to another by a sucking calf.

Clotted milk can indicate a staphylococcal, or streptococcal infection, or the severity of the infection. Strep & Staph infections are the most common types of mastitis in New Zealand.

Nature provides the udder, the teat, and the teat canal with protection from invading bacteria. But teats need care, so they can continue to be a barrier to micro-organisms.

Preventing Mastitis: Provide a stress free environment for milking.

Milking machines need care:

Cleanliness: Rinse after milking, and follow this by sanitizing the clusters pipes, & lines after use. "Detergents" are available from farm supply stores.

Machines Care: The pulsation, the vacuum, and cup liners are important. These influence the suction, or have contact with the teat. Machines need checking ideally 6 monthly. Faults need to be quickly fixed. By milking any mastitis cows last, you can avoid spreading the disease to other cows. Check on the mineral status of your animals.

Teat Spraying

The teat canal remains open for some time after milking..

Teat spraying with an antiseptic plus emollient solution (e.g. glycerine) immediately after milking will help prevent bacteria entering the teat canal. The addition of glycerine (or similar) enhances the teat's skin health. Use a sprayer that sprays upright, and aim at the teat opening. Then circle and spray so the sides of the teats also get a covering.

The antiseptic spray kills bacteria on the teat ends so they cannot enter the teat canal.

(Milkers can spray their hands with the solution also.) Mix up new solution of spray daily. Spray the teats throughout the milking season. *Spraying is preferable to dipping teats in a solution, or using a cloth. What happens in Mastitis:

Staphylococcal & streptococci mastitis is common in NZ. These bacteria invade the deeper parts of the gland.. To "fight" the invading bacteria, blood flow to the area increases, which produces the visible signs: heat & redness, swelling & a painful quarter. The small udder ducts can become blocked, and the affected alveoli will no longer produce milk.

Should the blockage become permanent, (and they can) this will stop antibiotics getting at the target. The bacteria remain, and are trapped inside like an abscess.

Some bacteria may leak, and infect other alveoli. She may also "leak" bacteria, and this can spread to other cows. These cases can be difficult to cure. Dry cow therapy is recommended.

E Coli Infections

E coli infections can be picked up from dung.. (Not so common in NZ.)

It is ideal to have cows calve in clean pasture, away from cow "camp sites" where they shelter, and "empty out" during bad weather. Signs and symptoms of an E coli infection vary dramatically. Some cows have enough defences (neutrophils) to kill the bacteria off quickly. But symptoms can range from a swollen painful quarter, to the animal being very ill. Call the vet if you have an ill feverish animal. She certainly won't be eating. The E coli releases toxins. Antibiotic treatment is usually started immediately.

Some quarters will need to be discontinued for the rest of the season, but they will return to milking the next season.

The RMT (Rapid mastitis test) or the Californian mastitis test.

Use a purchased reagent.. or just use the detergent you use for washing the dishes.

In a container.. add a squirt of cows milk from one quarter. Add a squirt of detergent to the milk. Swirl these fluids around.

If this mixture thickens you know you have a quarter with mastitis..

Clinical mastitis: This is the mastitis you have when the signs and symptoms are obvious.

Sub-clinical Mastitis: The signs are not obvious. The cow may have a high somatic cell count. In a RMT the combined milk and detergent will thicken. Early detection & fast action is needed when treating Mastitis.: The sooner antibiotic therapy is commenced the better the result. The vets will have a range of intra mammary antibiotics for sale. These will properly treat the known bacteria that are common in your geographical area.

You may be Faced with a Decision: Which intra-mammary to choose? There will be a price range. Some antibiotics have a different with holding period. The aim is to treat the infection quickly, with an antibiotic appropriate for the infection. (You can always take a sample of milk for culture & sensitivity prior to starting the antibiotic. It can be stored in the refrigerator for 24 hours.)

Administering an intra mammary "infusion":

Read the label on the container..Note: The withholding time. Write on your notes the animals identification and the day treatment commenced Milk the animal out first..

Gently cleans the end of the teat using cotton wool soaked with methylated spirits.

The tip of the antibiotic tube (once the cover is removed) is sterile.. Ensure it doesn't touch anything, and is inserted directly into the teat orifice... It can be a challenge with some animals!! Milk mastitis animals last. Identify the animal somehow as a "antibiotic cow" to minimise mistakes, (like the milk going into the vat.)and: Give the dose as stated..

There is no merit in doubling the dose. Sometimes there are advantages of administering an antibiotic injections as well as the intra-mammary infusion. Ask the vet about a suitable antibiotic to use. Use the same antibiotic for the course of the treatment.. Note the animals response.. If it is improving but clearly the infection is still there.. There may be merit in continuing for several days more. If there is no response to antibiotic treatment after several days, then use another antibiotic. BUT: Ask your vet for his/her advice.

Switching drugs can lead to bacterial resistance. (You cannot do a culture and sensitivity to see which antibiotic is most appropriate now..as the milk will have been contaminated by the 1st antibiotic you used.) Using dry cow at drying off is recommended for animals who have had clinical mastitis during the year..

Dry Cow Therapy: Giving "dry cow antibiotic's" immediately after the final milking of the season will help "clean up any infections" from the last milking season, and prevent infections during the dry period. Dry cow therapy is certainly recommended for cows who have had obvious infections during the milking season, and those with a high cell count.

The antibiotic is long acting.. it stays in the udder far longer.

Do not use on cows you are planning to cull.. it does have a much longer withholding period. Teat seal products are an option for cows with low cell counts, and who have NOT had mastitis. These products seal the teat orifice, preventing bacteria from entering.

Scouring, (fluid like faeces) Ill thrift, then rapid emaciation. It is fatal.

Onset: Some deer may exhibit the symptoms before 12 months old. Often stress will start the disease progressing. It may live in the animals body for years prior to the animal showing any symptoms. Spread: It is spread by infected faeces. Often calves and fawns pick it up from drinking from teats of infected mothers.

There is some possibility that it can spread to other young animals. Diagnosis, is by blood tests or faeces specimen. There *is no treatment*: The only way to deal with the disease is elimination of the animal with a positive blood or faeces test.

***Causes*:** It is an eye infection, but dust, bright sunlight, flies and irritation (e.g. thistles) may cause this condition. It is more common in summer and autumn. It can spread from one animal to another.

***Signs*:** 1st signs, tears streaming down the animals face. The animal blinks frequently, then signs of an infection appear. Untreated this can lead to permanent eye damage. **Note*: the animal may use only its 'good' eye (it will turn its head towards you). Its sore eye may be hidden from your view. If you notice one animal with pinkeye, check the rest of the group.

***Treatment*:** Antibiotic cream available from the vets. Apply as instructed.

Woody Tongue

***Appearance of Infected Animal*:** The soft tissues around the mouth, including the tongue are infected. The tongue becomes hard and swollen. The animal dribbles. They are reluctant to eat.

***What to Do*:** Observe the animal closely, then phone the vet, or speak to the vet. Describe the areas of swelling. He/she will prescribe a suitable antibiotic.

***Treatment*:** This disease responds well to the appropriate antibiotic. This infection appears from time to time. The organisms responsible are found in the soil.

About Antibiotics

Antibiotics Kill Only Bacteria: They do not kill viruses, or animal cells. Bacteria, are single cell organisms. Once they get past the animals immune system they rapidly reproduce causing disease.

Signs and Symptoms of Infection

This means the body is working to destroy infection.

Choice of Antibiotic: It is chosen because it is known to kill the bacteria causing a certain infection. e.g. bovine uterine infections: Tetracycline might be used.

Beware: Antibiotics can kill bacteria indiscriminately, e.g. the normal gut bacterial flora, which can happen if administering antibiotics to a young calf. Administer: The correct amount: (and for weight and age) the correct route, and the correct time, and for the prescribed length of time (e.g. 4 days).

Superbugs: If an animal has an adverse reaction to the antibiotic, do discontinue it. But: By not giving the antibiotic for the correct number of days. (regardless if the animals seems to have returned to health) Giving an incorrect doseage... you are contributing to a superbug existence. Superbugs *are bacteria which are resistant to nearly all antibiotics.* We use antibiotics so frequently, and now some bacteria simply won't be killed by some once-effective antibiotics. Culture and sensitivity: Together in conditions encouraging bacterial growth (culture) are bacteria, and samples of antibiotics. The bacterias response to the patches of antibiotic is observed. If there is no bacterial growth near a particular antibiotic sample It means the antibiotic is suitable for treating the disease... The bacteria is sensitive to that bacteria.

Vaccinations

Vaccinations prepare the immune system, so that the immunie systems are primed to kill off invading pathogenes. Some vaccinations are given in late pregnancy so the newborn has some immunity, or immunity is passed through colostrum e.g. rotovirus.

Inbreeding Depression

There is currently 1.5 to 1.8 million species in the world that have been successfully named and classified. Of this number a vast amount already has, or is in the process of extinction. Loss of habitat, over-exploitation of wildlife for commercial purposes, the introduction of harmful exotic species, environmental pollution, and the spread of diseases pose serious threats to the world's biological heritage. This is of key concern as the removal of a single species can set off a chain reaction in the ecosystem affecting many others. This is especially true for keystone species, whose loss can transform or undermine the ecological processes or fundamentally change the species composition of the wildlife community.

(U.S Fish And WildLife Service, 2005)Is there a method in which these species can be saved from extinction and reintroduced into the wildlife? A zoological garden shortened to zoo, is an institution in which animals are exhibited in captivity. In addition to providing visitors with an entertaining spectacle, modern zoos are also involved with conservation biology (PA, 2005). Conservation biology is the scientific study of the nature and status of the earth's biodiversity with the aim of protecting species, their habitats, and ecosystems from excessive rates of extinction (Soule, 1986).

Zoos meet there conservation role through captive breeding, the process of raising plants or animals in controlled conditions to produce stock for release into the wild, education, research, animal welfare, environmental enrichment, reintroduction and support for in situ conservation of species (F, 2008). Despite many efforts being made into conserving species, there are however some major constraints faced by zoos in meeting their conservation role while at the same time providing opportunities for the public to learn more about and enjoy nature in artificial forms. One major constraint faced by zoos, is the cost and time to conserve some species.

Large species breed at a much slower rates than other species and undergo seasonal breeding and require extensive fostering. An average cost of 1 million dollars in the USA is needed per year/per zoo. Therefore zoos require continued funds by tourism, and other methods in order to keep these species conserved. Other consequences arise within species themselves. Species that are kept conserved in zoos for a long period of time, result in a loss of behaviour in the wildlife, and essentially the species become adapted to zoo life.

Species that have been kept in zoos for a long period of time, are in the habit of extensive care and nourishment, and therefore become adapted to living in a predator free environment. However, when let out into the wild, these species have no experience in searching for food and avoiding predators therefore natural selection will select for these traits that are advantageous in captivity, but deleterious in the wild population.

A major approach that is taken to conserve an endangered species is inbreeding, which is breeding between closely related species, most often a result of population bottleneck. This is a major comeback for conservation as inbreeding often results to-inbreeding depression which is a reduction in the species fitness, and eventually leads to reductions in genetic variability.

In a population where inbreeding occurs most offspring's will have recessive deleterious traits and these traits will be masked by heterozygosity, and so natural selection will select against heterozygote's. (Lynch, 2005) Inbreeding depression is a major consequence of captive breeding, as seen in species such as Lion population, South China Tiger, and the California Condor. These are just a few out of the numerous numbers of endangered species, which have undergone captive breeding and have been made an attempt at to keep conserved in the wildlife population.

In order to illustrate the detrimental effects of Inbreeding depression, Packer et al, 1990 examined the declining lion population in Ngorongoro Crater which is an extinct volcanic caldera located at the western edge of the Gregory Rift. The lion population estimated to be at about 60 to 75 individuals over the period 1957-1961. In 1962 however, the lion population suffered an extraordinary outbreak of Stomoxys calcitrans biting flies that reduced the population to about nine females and one male. (C.Packer, 1991) Because of the drastic reduction in population size, there was extensive inbreeding amongst the survivor species. As examined by Packer et al, 1990 Ngorongoro Crater was largely repopulated by descendents of a group of four females.

Each successive cohort of cubs belonging to these four females subsequently became established breeders and mated with only seven breeding males that immigrated to the Crater all during the period shortly after the outbreak. However once the surviving females had bred successfully, the large coalitions of males prevented any further immigration which further increased inbreeding and therefore levels of heterozygosity subsequently declined by 10 percent. With a decline in levels of heterozygosity there is evidence that shows impaired reproduction in the Crater lions and higher proportion of abnormal sperm, which reduces sperm quality such that it penetrates female eggs at a very low rate. As a result productivity of the Crate population has declined since the 1970's and as predicted the average levels of heterozygosity in this population will continue to decline in the future in the absence of any male immigration.

A similar study of a lion species named Panthera Leo, abundant in Africa suffered population bottle neck due to loss of habitat. (Bjorklund, 2003) And this resulted in reduced genetic diversity which is correlated with reduction in survival. This results in a higher population decline and can increase the rate of extinction.

Therefore, as demonstrated by Packer et al, and Bjorklund et al, reduction in population size of a species promotes inbreeding which causes a decline in genetic diversity, and ultimately has detrimental effects on the species.

Inbreeding depression has also been observed in the South China tiger, by study done by (Y.C. et al, 2007). The South China Tiger (Panthera Tigris Amoyensis) is a subspecies of tiger native to forests of southern China. Of the currently present 5 tiger species, the South China Tiger is the rarest and the most critically endangered due to factors including hunting, poaching and habitat loss. However one of the most serious threats to tiger's survival is the use of tiger products in traditional Chinese medicines. The tiger bone is considered to be one of the most valued as a treatment to various conditions. (Tilson, 1997) Due to these factors the individuals declined from a reputed number of 4000 species in 1950's and continued to decline until the mid 1990's when the number of free ranging species was estimated to be fewer than 20 individuals (Gilson et al.2004).

In the 1950's however four females and two males were captured from the wild and were used to found a captive population. (Y.C.Xu, 2007). Because of the vast decrease in population number, the 6 founder population were enforced to inbreed in the 1970's and continues to inbreed because of comeback such as their mating behaviour. Female tigers can only mate when they reach maturity at 3 years of age and only in temperate climates seasonally. Because of this only a small number of tigers are able to breed in each generation which lead to inbreeding depression in 1972. As observed by (Y.C.XU et al, 2007) inbreeding depression in the population shows low level of juvenile survivorship due to the loss of genetic variation and because of this infants were not able to adjust to the changing environmental conditions. Also because of low fertility and fecundity, reproductive difficulties were observed amongst the species. As a result the small number of founders and inbreeding depression contribute to a major challenge of conserving the South China Tiger.

Inbreeding depression has also occurred in the wild population of the California Condor that ranged from British Columbia to Baja

California in the 19th century (Vickey, 2000). During that time period, the species faced dramatic population decline caused by high mortality rates due to exploitation, habitat destruction and the most prominent factor lead poisoning.

It wasn't until the 1987, that all the remaining population of 27 individuals of which 14 were males and 13 are females were captured and brought into captivity. (Phillip, 1995) Due to the small population size, there was extensive inbreeding which led to the loss of genetic variation and changes in allele frequency. The population also harvested a vast amount of deleterious recessive alleles, which are usually depleted of the population by natural selection. Before the decline in the Condor population there is much genetic variability, and therefore recessive deleterious alleles are hidden from natural selection by dominant alleles.

However when the population declined, and inbreeding was enforced, close relatives that mate one another likely carry the same recessive deleterious alleles. Accordingly when relatives mate the offspring may inherit two copies of the same recessive deleterious allele expressing it. According to the study conducted by (Ralls et al. 1999), captive flocks had produced five deformed embryos that exhibited Chondrodystrophy, and died near the time of hatching. Chondrodystrophy, a recessive deleterious allele in chickens, is a condition where the abnormal development of cartilage affects bone growth before birth, and eventually leads to dwarfism. Chondrodystrophy in birds can be caused by a variety of factors such as mycoplasma infections and dietary deficiencies, particularly of manganese. (Ralls et al. 1999). Therefore inbreeding depression exposes Chondrodystrophy in offspring's, which results in a high mortality rate and ultimately reduction in population and stability of species extinction.

Other species that are affected by recessive deleterious alleles caused by inbreeding are Golden Lion Tamarin's (Leontopithecus rosalia). According to study done by (Bush et al. 1996), Golden Lion Tamarin's are native to the forests of Brazil and are widely endangered with a captive population originating in 1982 due to extensive deforestation. The current captive population of 494 individuals underwent inbreeding, which resulted Diaphragmatic defects, a disease caused by recessive deleterious alleles. A diaphragmatic defect is a rare syndrome characterised mainly by a defect in the diaphragm that allows some of the abdominal organs to move into the chest cavity, and involved missing or formation of abnormal bones in the arms or legs. (M., 1980) Therefore inbreeding depression was observable in the Lion population and posed major consequences.

As seen in the California Condor and Golden Lion Tamarin, low genetic diversity caused by reduction in population will result in inbreeding depression. This will unmask of recessive deleterious alleles in the offspring's of the parental generation, and will result in the depletion of these individuals due to natural selection.

Today, more species are alive on the planet than ever before. Estimates place the number of species between 10 to 100 million, with only 1.5 to 1.8 million identified with Latin names (Lacy, 1997). Of this number studies indicate that 2 to 3 species are going extinct yearly due to a wide number of reasons such as exploitation, habitat destruction, pollution, global warming, introduction of exotic species, and the spread of diseases. Why should we initially care about species going extinct?

Major concern isn't about extinction of a single species, but rather the ecosystem it belongs to, and the interaction with other species. Some species play a vital role in there ecosystem, that if lost due to extinction, it could affect a numerous number of species. Zoos across the world now hold a major role in conserving these species. Species that are headed towards extinction are captured from the wild and placed in zoos in which they are provided an artificial habitat much like their own. With the rather small population of species, professionals employ captive breeding amongst them.

It is the process of capturing animals from the wild and mating them in captivity in order to increase the number of species under protected conditions. (Waugh, 1988) Despite many species that have been reintroduced into the wild as a result of captive breeding, there is a downfall. Firstly, captive breeding programs focuses only on a few charismatic endangered species, and neglects the numerous number of other species that are in the process of extinction. It is also very costly to train individuals to capture species from the wild, and provide them with their mimicry habitat and other resources they require.

A major consequence faced by conservation however, is inbreeding depression seen in species that mate relatives, or siblings. Major consequences of Inbreeding depression are seen in the Lion population, South China Tiger, and California Condor. Because of their relatively small population due to factors such as habitat destruction, these species were captured from the wild, and had gone through inbreeding.

A major consequence of inbreeding is the reduction in fitness and the loss of genetic diversity. As the closely related species kept on inbreeding within themselves, it was only those alleles that were being expressed. With a loss of genetic diversity, offspring's of those individuals are not able to withstand the changing environment. Other consequences of inbreeding seen in California Condor, is the expressivity of a recessive deleterious allele. The offspring's exhibited diseases caused by these recessive alleles.

Hence, when a population undergoes a bottleneck affect, most zoos try a technique commonly knows as inbreeding to try and preserve a species. Inbreeding also has its consequences as it is apparent in the three species discussed above. The most direct effect of inbreeding is inbreeding depression as it causes a reduction in population number.

Transgenic Mammals and Gene Targeting

Transgenic Mammals and Gene Targeting-Biology Research Paper

Molecular biotechnology has been one of the most prospective fields of science for more than three decades. Its applications are numerous and have not even come close to reaching the limit. Since discovery of genes scientists have been researching a way to temper with them to achieve a desirable effect. In last two decades technology became available which allows introduction of specific genetic material from a donor into a host organism. Organisms which have altered or foreign genetic material, are now being referred to as transgenic. (Wang, 2003) Several methods have been devised for introduction or modification of genetic material. Most common and most controversial is embryonic stem-cell mediated gene transfer. It involves introduction of modified DNA into embryonic stem-cells, which will take up the DNA and hopefully express the desired genes. Application of this kind of technology is practically limitless. It scope spans across multiple industries, varying from agricultural uses to medical applications. (Westphal, 1989)

Latest achievements involve production of medically important proteins like anti-clotting factors through expression of the gene in lactating cows, goats and pigs. (William 1997)

Industries like agriculture have been desperate to express desired traits in livestock in order to increase production and the quality of the product in order to meet the demand of growing population. The most common fields in transgenic livestock that are being researched are: growth, pathogen resistance and quality of meat products. Many more applications of transgenic technology are now being considered as the field expands almost exponentially.

However the most important application of this technology so far is identification of gene function. Function of the gene can be found by "turning it off" and studying the effect on the organism. This approach is known as gene targeting or gene knockout. (Capecchi, 1994)

Background

Genomes of several mammals have been sequenced so far and few more are under way. Knowing the base pair composition of the genome is only half the task done, the other half would be the identification of gene function. Most common genes are present in all species, thus they are identified with relative ease. Genes that are completely unknown are much harder to identify as very little is known about them. Gene targeting is a most common technique being used to identify the function of the gene.

It involves introduction of a mutation into the "unknown" gene which will suppress its expression. Usually it is a mutation of the start codon or promoter region, however many more possibilities are available. The genome with inactivated gene is introduced into embryo and then selected for. Embryo that has taken up the DNA is then introduced into surrogate mother who will give berth to a transgenic offspring. Offspring is then mated with each other in order to create a homozygote of the mutation. Homozygotes are then studied for the effect of the mutation on the functioning of the organism. (Capecchi, 1994)

DNA microinjections is a common technique used for gene targeting as it involves manipulation and reintroduction of the genetic material into the same species.

Many genes have been identified through loss of function. For example, recently it was found that a transcription factor is responsible for mammalian cold sensation. Transgenic mice that were created that had a mutation in the gene which codes for the transcription factor (NGFIB). They were unable to respond to cold stimuli which provided strong evidence that a transcription factor is indeed required in the cold response pathway. (Kim, 2005)

A discrepancy in the metabolic pathway of the organism would indicate that a gene coding for a "missing factor" isn't functioning thus will allow its isolation and identification.

Major Topic

First transgenic experiments were carried out on mice. In 1981 first transgenic mammal was created. The animal had a copy of human growth hormone integrated into its genome. It was hypothesized that a growth hormone gene would speed up and increase overall growth of the mice. The outcome was as expected, a mouse which grew quicker and was much bigger in size.

Today application of the technology is expanding. Human growth hormone was also introduced to pigs. (Westphal, 1989) The experiment was a success as produced pigs had larger carcasses and less body fat. However there was a downside to the outcome, transgenic pigs were infertile. However research is being carried out to solve the infertility problem. There also was a huge public opinion formed on transgenic animals. Public view of transgenic animals is that they maybe harmful to both humans and the environment. Some critics say that scientist accelerate "selection" through transgenic technologies. In the end all comes down to ethics, which will have a final word on use of transgenic animals.

One aspect of technology that have bypassed both ethics and public opinion was use of transgenic mice of identify unknown genes. Mice are perfect for study of gene function. They have high reproduction rate, a lot is known about mouse genome and they are relatively easy to handle.

Gene targeting allowed identification of the function of genes which were previously unknown. In early 1990s research was conducted on function of Insulin-like growth factors. Knockout mice were created with a mutation in the insulin-like growth factor gene. Produced mice showed delayed bone development, retarded post-natal growth, growth deficiency and infertility. (FBS) Hence it proved that insulin-like growth factor plays an important role in fetal development. (DeChiara, 1990; Baker J, 1993) IGF2 gene is located on chromosome 11, p15.5 in mice. Further knockout experiments proved that IGF2 is jointly regulated with H19 and INS2 genes and all theses genes play vital role in fetal development. (Strachan, T 1999)

In 2004 group of Japanese and Korean scientist were successful in creating a parthenogenetic mice which survived and grew into adulthood. They were successful through careful manipulation of IGF2, H19 and INS2 genes. These genes are imprinted during early embryonic development as on copy comes from a father and one from a mother. Through manual imprinting of the gene (introduction of the deletion in the promoter region) in prepared oocyte, they were successful in creating an offspring without a physical father. (Kono, 2004)

This emphasizes the result gene knockout technique can have on the outcome of the study. Knowledge of a single gene function contributed to discovery which had a world wide impact.

Discussion

Transgenic animals so far have proven to benefit humanity in every way. Medical applications have proved to be a great benefit and thus created a positive public opinion. On other hand use of transgenic animals in agriculture is considered dangerous to us and the environment. Agricultural applications of transgenic animals would be a great asset to the industry as costs will be cut and product produced will have higher quality. Industrial uses are not under direct criticism as they are mostly controlled by the private sector. The private applications are have lesser exposure. For example in Canada, scientists in private sector have introduced silk spider genes into lactating goats. The experiment was a success as goats were producing silk from mammary glands. The company, Nexia Biotechnologies also has claimed that they are aiming to produce other industrially important products from lactating goats (Nexia).

General public doesn't really have an opinion on use of this controversial technology as its opinion is force fed by individuals who obviously don't like the idea. Many topics have been brought up as scientists and governments have made ground rules on what is allowed and what's not. Topics like ethics, morals, god and human responsibility as only morally capable and accountable creatures on this planet have been the major weapon of hypocrites against technology that will be saving lives and providing us with better quality products at reduced cost. (Outka, 2002)

Future applications of the technology would range from production of important proteins to release of wide range of transgenic farming animals. Research is being carried out on pigs to create spare organs that will be compatible with human physiology. Research is also underway to manufacture milk through transgenesis for treatment of debilitating diseases such as phenylketonuria (PKU), hereditary emphysema, and cystic fibrosis. (Margawati, 2003)

Conclusion

Insertion or manipulation of genetic material is a system that gives rise to transgenic animals. Several methods have been devised for introduction of the genetic material into the host. Most commonly DNA is directly inserted into the pronuclei of the egg through the technique called microinjection. The following egg is introduced into the surrogate mother. Identification of the offspring that have taken up the DNA is a next logical step. (Capecchi, 1994) Using the following technique scientists have been able to create "super" animals which have traits that are superior to other animals.

The technology has unlimited amount of applications in fields of medicine, agriculture and industrial biotechnology. Transgenic mammals are widely found in agriculture where traits like increased carcass size, product quality and disease resistance are in high demand. Medical applications of the technology involve production of proteins which are essential for survival of people with blood clotting disorders. (Westphal, 1989)

Identification of gene function is probably the most important exploit of the transgenic technology. Genomes of several animals have been successfully sequenced, but function of the identified genes is at most a guess. Gene targeting is a technique in which the gene under question is disabled through various means and then introduced into the pronucleus of the egg. The egg is then inserted into surrogate mother who will hopefully give birth to the offspring lacking the functional gene. The identified mutant is then studied, whether it's looking for discrepancy in the metabolic pathway or the gene end product. (Capecchi, 1994)

Mice have been used extensively in gene targeting as they produce a lot of progeny, easy to maintain and handle. Today many previously unknown genes have been identified using gene targeting technique. Technology is on the rise as more genomes are being sequenced and more genes are found. Uses of transgenic animals are vast and are proving to benefit the humanity greatly.

Bracken Poisoning in Cattle

Many plant poisonings, including bracken poisoning, are common in the autumn. The highest risk period is when grass growth is poor, particularly if this has been combined with bracken control so that rhizomes or new young fronds are available for cattle to eat.

Bracken contains a variety of toxins. For cattle the two most important are a toxin that depresses the bone marrow, and a cancer–causing toxin. These toxins are still active in hay made from pastures with bracken

Clinical Signs—Acute Poisoning

This occurs as a result of eating large quantities of bracken. Disease develops because of depression of the bone marrow, which stops the production of the white cells that fight infection and the platelets that help blood to clot. Signs can up to eight weeks after cattle have stopped eating bracken

- Depression and loss of appetite
- Bloody diarrhoea accompanied by straining
- High temperature
- Bleeding from nose, eyes and vagina
- Weakening, collapse and death (usually within five days of the onset of signs)
- Secondary infection is very common.

Enzootic Haematuria

This occurs as the result of eating small quantities of bracken over a long period of time. Cancerous changes occur in the bladder leading to:

- In mild cases-persistently bloody urine (haematuria)
- In severe cases – severe blood loss and difficulty passing urine with visible blood clots

In some animals, cancer occurs in the gut as well as the bladder. The signs depend on the site of the tumour. Get veterinary advice in animals showing unusual gut signs that have had access to bracken

Diagnosis

- On the clinical signs described above
- History of access to bracken
- Blood sample for haematology
- In many cases a post mortem will be essential to confirm the diagnosis.

Treatment

- There is no specific antidote for bracken poisoning.
- Broad-spectrum antibiotics to prevent secondary infection can help in acute cases
- For animals with haematuria no treatment is effective.

Prevention

1. Limit access to pastures with bracken, particularly if grazing is poor
2. Never allow cattle access to recently ploughed land where bracken has been. Exposed rhizomes are the most dangerous part of the plant as they are attractive to cattle. Particularly if they have started to reshoot
3. Bracken control by burning, ploughing, reseeding, and herbicide is the best method of prevention.

Poisonous Plants

Plant poisoning is nationally important to Australia. About a thousand species of plants here are known to be toxic to livestock and humans. Poisoning of livestock by the more important of these costs us about $100 million each year. Deaths of cattle from plant poisoning in Queensland cost over $10 million yearly.

Sixty percent of the toxic plants in Australia are native to this country and have their major economic effect on agricultural enterprises which produce livestock by grazing native pastures. These industries contribute significantly to export-generated income and thus to our prosperity as a nation. This makes the reduction of the effects of plant poisoning on livestock one of the serious concerns of the pastoral industries.

The toxic native species belong to about 70 of the over 200 native plant families in Australia. Families with more than 10 toxic species include the legumes (Fabaceae, Mimosaceae), the nightshades and tobaccos (Solanaceae), the spurges (Euphorbiaceae), the grasses (Poaceae), the cycads (Cycadaceae, Zamiaceae), the saltbushes (Chenopodiaceae), the riceflowers (Thymelaeaceae) and the buttercups (Ranunculaceae). Some genera are generally toxic (for example *Macrozamia* and *Pimelea*), but it is important to note that a number of important toxic species (for example *Erythrophleum chlorostachys* and *Trema tomentosa*) have few or no known toxic relatives.

What is a Poisonous Plant?

Poisonous plants broadly include members of the cyanobacteria (blue-green algae), fungi, ferns, cone-bearing and flowering plants. They are understood by most people to be those which cause disease in humans or domestic animals after being eaten. This is quite true from the medical and veterinary viewpoint, but not really so when the whole spectrum of animal-plant interaction is considered. Strictly, if a plant is to be defined as poisonous, the animals that are susceptible to the toxin or toxins in the plant should be defined as well. For example, the nectar of *Lomatia silaifolia* flowers contains cyanide and is reputed to kill flies, but is not known to poison livestock. Conversely, I have seen beetle larvae feeding on the fronds of *Cycas armstrongii* which would be fatal for cattle.

Whether a plant is poisonous or not depends on the capacity of the animal eating it to cope with the chemicals it contains. The outcome of eating such plants may be further complicated if the concentration of their toxins varies with the stage of growth of the plants or the seasonal conditions, rendering the plant more hazardous at some times than at others.

What Do Poisonous Plants Look Like?

There are no common characteristics of form, colouring, odour or taste which distinguish a poisonous plant from a non-poisonous plant. To avoid poisoning, we need to learn what the known poisonous plants look like, based on the knowledge generated by past experience and scientific studies of the subject. The books of Everist, McBarron and Dowling and McKenzie can help with the recognition of poisonous plants in Australia.

Why are Plants Poisonous?

Current opinion appears to be that many of the plant chemicals toxic to humans and livestock are produced as part of the plant's defences against being eaten or to gain an advantage over competing plants. Many of these defences are directed against insects. This makes the poisoning of people and their animals truly "accidental" and "collateral damage" in the long wars between plant and plant and between plants and the insects which eat them.

The known plant toxins are part of a group of chemicals known as secondary compounds or metabolites because they are not essential to the basic bio-chemistry of the plants. They include such things as waste products, storage products and flower pigments as well as growth inhibitors and toxins against predators. The caboxyatractylosides in noogoora burr (*Xanthium pungens*) seeds probably function to inhibit the growth of other plants which may compete with young burrs. These toxins will severely damage the liver of animals which eat them. They are also found in the native *Wedelia asperrima* which is known to poison sheep in northern Queensland. The cyanogenic glycosides in many plants including native or spotted fuchsia (*Eremophila maculata*) and native birdsfoot trefoil (*Lotus australis*) liberate cyanide when the plant tissue is damaged and kill insects, snails or slugs feeding on them. The same process may kill domestic animals as well.

Are Native Animals Poisoned?

Under normal circumstances, plant-eaters (including mammals and insects) have developed ways of avoiding being poisoned. These mechanisms are through modified behaviour and through chemical-based defences. Certain insects have developed to a point where plant toxins form part of their own defence, thus turning a hazard into an asset. The classic example of this is the association of milkweeds (*Asclepias curassavica*) with monarch butterflies whose larvae store the bitter and toxic cardiac glycosides from the plant. This deters birds from feeding on the caterpillars.

Generally, insects eat only one or a limited range of plant species and have developed specific chemical means of dealing with the toxic compounds in those plants. In contrast, mammalian plant-eaters generally use a wider range of plants and depend on taste, smell and learning to avoid toxic species.

They have more broadly-based chemical detoxication systems in the chemical mechanisms of their livers and other organs and in the microbes in their stomachs and intestines.

A good example of the adaption of mammals to a plant toxin by developing an efficient chemical detoxication method in the liver is the interaction of some Western Australian animals with many fluoroacetate-containing plants (*Gastrolobium* species) in the south-western part of the state. Brush-tailed possums, bush rats and western grey kangaroos from this area are capable of safely eating these plants which are rapidly fatal for livestock, red kangaroos, eastern grey kangaroos and for brush-tailed possums and bush rats from eastern Australia. *Gastrolobium grandiflorum* and *Acacia georginae*, which grow in Queensland, also contain this toxin which is the toxic component of 1080 poison.

Because plant-eaters are well adapted to their natural environments, poisoning occurs only when those environments are seriously disturbed (for example by drought or human interference) and animals are forced to leave their accustomed ecological niches to feed on dangerous plants. Koalas are believed to have been poisoned by cyanide while feeding on fresh young regrowth of manna gums (*Eucalyptus viminalis*) after bushfires in Victoria.

Perhaps the ultimate in forcing animals out of their ecological niches was the introduction of European farm animals and humans to the totally new plants of Australia and other European colonies in the Americas and southern Africa.

A Little Australian History

The first plant poisonings in eastern Australia recorded by Europeans were suffered by the people and pigs of Cook's expedition of 1770 while they were repairing HMS Endeavour at the mouth of the Endeavour River in northern Queensland. Joseph Bank's journal describes the plant and its effects. The seeds of *Cycas media* seem to be the most likely cause of the diarrhoea and vomiting among the men and death in some of the pigs. In the previous century, Dutch explorers of south-western Australia had similar experiences with the seeds of the cycad *Macrozamia riedlei.*

The first human inhabitants of Australia 40,000 years ago may have had similar experiences initially, but they learned to extract the toxins from the seeds of *Cycas* and *Macrozamia* species. By about 4000 years ago, they were using the resulting food to support large gatherings of people for ceremonies in Arnhem Land and in the Carnarvon Ranges of central Queensland. The known chemical compounds in untreated cycad seeds are not actually toxic themselves but need modification by bacteria in the intestines to yield the toxin methylazoxymethanol (MAM) which is a potent cancer-producer and causes liver damage. The toxin which causes spinal cord damage in cattle which eat cycad leaves is not known.

Another food plant of the original Australians and described near Brisbane by Alan Cunningham on expedition in 1828 and 1829 was the Moreton Bay chestnut or black bean (*Castanospermum australe*). Its seeds, toxic when raw, were prepared by roasting or soaking in water.

Few European overland explorers of Australia suffered from plant poisoning, but some are recorded. During the 1864-65 journey of the Jardine brothers from Rockhampton to Cape York, 30 of their 42 horses and 50 of their 250 cattle died after eating a poisonous plant near the Wenlock River on Cape York peninsula. It seems likely that the plant involved was the Cooktown ironwood (*Erythrophleum chlorostachys*) which is common in tropical Australia and highly toxic to livestock. Ernest Giles reported the death of two of his camels and illness of others after eating *Gyrostemon ramulosus* (sandhill corkbark, camel poison) during his central Australian expeditions of 1875-76.

Once the pastoral invasion of Australia began in earnest, many thousands of domestic grazing animals were poisoned by native plants to which they were unadapted.

A Posy of Native Poisonous Plants

The following is a mixed bouquet of toxic native flowering plants (with some greenery!), not mentioned elsewhere in this article. Some of these may find their way into our gardens. Some certainly deserve to do so as very attractive specimens.

Pimelea species in eastern Australia have been recognised for some time as the cause of a serious disease of cattle which produces anaemia, diarrhoea and heart failure with spectacular fluid accumulations under the skin. The plants involved are usually *Pimelea trichostachya, P. simplex* or *P. elongata*, collectively known as flaxweeds. The toxins in these plants are particularly irritant and probably occur in most, if not all, *Pimelea* species. Two other toxic species in Queensland are rather attractive red-flowered *P. haematostachya* and *P. decora*.

Certain ferns contain important toxins. Bracken (*Pteridium esculentum, Pteridium revolutum*) and mulga or rock fern (*Cheilanthes sieberi*) contain ptaquiloside which damages the bone marrow of cattle when taken in large amounts and produces bladder cancer in cattle when eaten in small amounts over several years. These ferns and nardoo (*Marsilea drummondii*) contain on enzyme which destroy vitamin B1, leading to brain damage in sheep and horses. You may recall that Bourke and Wills were fed nardoo cakes made from the ground sporocarps by their aboriginal rescuers near Cooper's Creek. It has been thought that their subsequent deaths may have been related to the toxin in nardoo, but this seems very unlikely. *Bowenia serrulata*, known as Byfield fern but in fact a cycad, has poisoned cattle in the same way that other cycads in Australia have.

Two rainforest trees whose fruits have poisoned children are white cedar (*Melia azedarach* var. *australasica*) and finger cherry (*Rhodomyrtus macrocarpa*). Finger cherry fruit were associated with cases of permanent blindness in northern Queensland in the first half of this century. The stage at which the fruit are dangerous is unclear. Prudence suggests that they should not be eaten at all, but the local aboriginal people have used them as a food source. The details of poisoning of children by white cedar fruits are even more vague, but pigs are occasionally poisoned and have damage to their brains and intestines as the main effects.

The seeds of *Abrus precatorius* are highly toxic, but the seed coat is very hard and seeds swallowed intact pass through the gut without any ill effect. Immature seeds or those with a cracked seed coat will release toxin. One seed contains enough toxin to kill an adult human. There is severe damage to the stomach and intestines and other body systems.

Anthocercis viscosa (sticky tail flower) from the Albany region of Western Australia is reputed to be toxic to sheep, but evidence is scanty. *Anthocercis littorea* (yellow tail flower) is also suspected of poisoning. The fruits of this species have poisoned children in Western Australia.

Bottle trees (*Brachychiton rupestris*) have been known to poison cattle when felled and the pith of the trunk has been made available for drought feeding. The nitrate accumulated in this material has proved toxic.

The rattlepods (*Crotalaria* species) are a group of plants which contain pyrrolizidine alkaloids. These toxins accumulate in the liver and produce long-term damage which is often fatal. Horses and cattle are more susceptible to poisoning than sheep, but sheep have been poisoned by bluebush pea (*Crotalaria eremea* ssp. *eremea*) in western Queensland. Poisoned horses develop a condition called "walk-about disease" or "Kimberley horse disease" in which they become unaware of their surroundings and wander blindly. A major cause of this poisoning is *Crotalaria crispata*, a small plant common in the Kimberley region of Western Australia. Other *Crotalaria* species cause the disease in the remainder of tropical Australia. Recently, cattle in central Queensland have been poisoned by another plant containing these toxins, the variable groundsel or fireweed (*Senecio lautus*). Cattle with this long-term liver disease gradually lose weight and die.

In central and northern Queensland an unusual disease of horses is caused by two other species of *Crotalaria*, *C. aridicola* (Chillagoe horse poison) and *C. medicaginea* (trefoil rattlepod). Horses may develop a taste for these plants which damage the oesophagus (gullet) producing ulceration severe enough to stop the horse swallowing food.

Butterfly flag (*Diplarrena moraea*) from Tasmania and south-eastern mainland Australia and Morgan flower (*Morgania floribunda*) from drier parts of mainland Australia probably contain cardiac glycosides, the toxins in foxgloves (*Digitalis purpurea*) and cane toads (*Bufo marinus*). They have poisoned sheep and cattle, producing severe diarrhoea.

Waxflower (*Hoya australis*) growing in the softwood scrubs of Queensland has been used as a drought fodder for cattle. Too much will damage spinal cord function and cattle will collapse and may die.

Nervous system damage of a more severe kind in cattle enabled the rediscovery of a rare rainforest tree, *Idiospermum australiense*, in northern Queensland. Its seeds were found in the stomach contents of cattle which had died rapidly after feeding beneath the trees in 1971. The toxin responsible is unknown, but may be related to strychnine.

Nervous derangement is also a feature of Weir vine (*Ipomoea* sp. aff. *calobra*) poisoning of sheep in the Maranoa district of Queensland and caustic vine (*Sarcostemma brevipedicellatum*-formerly *S. australe*) poisoning of sheep in inland Queensland. Sheep are also the victims of muscle degeneration produced by eating the mature seed heads of the plains plover daisy or flat billy buttons (*Ixiolaena brevicompta*).

Selenium poisoning of horses leading to hoof deformation and loss of hair from the mane and tail has been associated with eating mapoon or ada-a (*Morinda reticulata*) on Cape York peninsula or *Neptunia amplexicaulis* in the Flinders River region of northern Queensland. Cattle and sheep may also be poisoned.

Ellangowan poison bush (*Myoporum deserti*) is one of a number of plants in Australia, native and exotic, which cause severe liver damage to cattle and sheep. Stock travelling on foot are most at risk. This is also the circumstance which leads to poisoning by the native tobaccos (*Nicotiana* species). They contain nicotine alkaloids and produce nervous system malfunction.

Irritation of the intestines leading to diarrhoea is a common consequence of plant poisoning and is reported in cattle after eating woolly waterlily or frogsmouth (*Philydrum lanuginosum*), native leek (*Bulbine bulbosa*) and buttercups of various sorts (*Ranunculus* species). Diarrhoea is a major sign of poisoning of cattle by Thargomindah nightshade (*Solanum sturtianum*). While all *Solanum* species are often regarded as potentially toxic, in reality only a small number of them have been demonstrated to be poisonous under field conditions.

Congenital defects can be caused by eating poisonous plants. Wild parsnips (*Trachymene ochracea, T. cyanantha* and *T.glaucifolia*) have been associated with "bentleg" of lambs after pregnant ewes grazed on these plants in western Queensland and north-western NSW.

Blindness of sheep and goats has followed their eating of nodding blue lily or blind grass (*Stypandra glauca*-known as *S.imbricata* and

S.grandiflora in Western Australia). Degeneration of the nerves connecting the eyes to the brain occurs. The toxin has been identified and is also present in smaller amounts in the blue flax lily (*Dianella revoluta*), but this plant has not been recorded as having caused poisoning.

Nervous system malfunction is seen in poisoning of livestock by some Darling peas (*Swainsona* species) and of cattle by some grasstrees (*Xanthorrhoea* species). *Swainsona galagifolia* is a common source of poisoning in eastern Australia, sheep being the most common victims. In Western Australia, *Swainsona canescens* is a common toxic species. Sheep are thought to develop a liking for these plants and may seek them out in the presence of other non-toxic feed. Cattle poisoned by grasstrees develop a disease called "wamps", a name derived form the sound made when an affected animal falls heavily to the ground. The grasstree most likely to be involved are *X fulva* (swamp grasstree) and *X.johnsonii* (northern forest grasstree).

Should We Grow Native Poisonous Plants in Our Gardens?

Why do we grow plants in our gardens? Some of the more important reasons include the pleasure we get from the appearance or fragrance of plants, their use as food and their capacity to improve the physical conditions in our homes by shading, boosting humidity, moderating wind and providing privacy. Unless the toxic plants which we may grow are likely to be eaten in dangerous amounts by susceptible individuals (usually young children or domestic animals), no hazard exists and we can enjoy their benefits in the same way as for any other garden plant. As a general rule, it would be wise to check the toxic properties of all your garden plants in the appropriate reference books. Prevention is certainly far more certain than cure for plants poisoning.

Poisonous Plants and Plant Toxins

Poisonous plants and other plant toxins are a major cause of economic loss the sheep and goat industry. Many cases of plant poisonings are never diagnosed or suspected. On this page, links are arranged alphabetically according to topic or toxicity:

Chapter 2

Some Plants of Kentucky Poisonous to Livestock

Poisonous plants are responsible for considerable losses to farmers and stockmen in Kentucky. Many cases of plant poisoning are never diagnosed or even suspected. There are nearly 100 different species of plants growing in Kentucky that under certain conditions may be poisonous to livestock. Only one third of these are likely to cause serious trouble. The primary purpose of this circular is to enable the farmer to recognise, at sight, plants which are known to be dangerously poisonous, and to have some knowledge of those additional plants, which, under certain conditions, may cause trouble.

Recognition of Plant Poisoning

Plant poisoning is often difficult to diagnose, since the symptoms vary with the plant eaten and the poisonous substances it contains. When plant poisoning is suspected, first eliminate the possibility that the animal is suffering from some infectious disease or chemical poisoning from paint, sprays or weed killers left around the farm. Plant poisoning may be suspected when there is a sudden onset of unexplained illness, acute disorders of the nervous system or the digestive tract, loss of weight, difficult breathing, weakness, coma and collapse. There is usually no fever, except in cases of poisoning by dogbanes and bracken. If the animal dies, autopsy finding of identifiable parts of poisonous plants in the animal's digestive tract may lead to a definite diagnosis.

Call a Veterinarian

When plant poisoning in livestock is recognised or suspected, the first thing to do is call a veterinarian, since diagnosis and treatment of a poisoned animal must be done early if the animal is to be saved. Some first aid can be given before the veterinarian arrives. Place the affected animal where it is quiet and comfortable and where diagnosis can be made and treatment given. The treatment will be determined by observing the series of symptoms, and finding what poisonous plant was eaten. Other livestock should not be allowed in the pasture where the poisoning occurred nor fed questionable silage or hay until the cause of the poisoning has been determined.

How to Prevent Plant Poisoning?

Learn to recognise poisonous plants. Study the illustrations and descriptions in this circular until you are familiar with them. Make a thorough survey of your property, wherever stock is turned out to graze. Poisonous plants sometimes occur in the open pasture, but more frequently along fence rows, banks of streams and ponds, and in woodlands. Learn to recognise these plants in their early stages of growth. Cockleburs and some others are poisonous only as seedlings. Send to the Agricultural Experiment Station, University of Kentucky, Lexington, Ky. 40506 for identification any plant that you cannot positively identify, but suspect to be poisonous.

Don't harvest poisonous plants in hay. Before hay is cut, the field should be carefully examined.

Avoid overgrazing. Most cases of plant poisoning are closely connected with a lack of suitable forage. When plenty of grass or hay is available, animals will usually avoid poisonous plants, which are often tough and unpalatable. Larkspur, dutchman's breeches, water hemlock and poison hemlock are particularly dangerous in the early spring. Likewise in the fall, when pastures are dry, animals will eat whatever is available, even trees and shrubs.

Suggestions for Sending Plant Specimens for Identification

Plants suspected of being poisonous may be sent for identification to the Department of Agronomy, Agricultural Science Building, Lexington, Kentucky.

When possible, send the entire plant, including leaves, flowers, roots, fruits, and seeds.

State the general structure or size of the plant, whether herb, shrub, tree or vine, colour of flowers, and locality and county where the plant was collected.

If two or more kinds of plants are sent at the same time, each plant should have a numbered tag attached to it. Fresh specimens should be wrapped in damp paper before mailing.

If plants cannot be sent in fresh condition, they should be pressed out flat and packed between pieces of cardboard before sending.

Description

Shoots round, hollow, jointed, of two types, arising from a perennial, creeping, underground rootstock. One type of shoot, tan in colour, appears in early spring, and bears the reproductive spores in a terminal, cone-like structure. The other is sterile and appears later, bearing whorls of pine-needle-like branches. Leaves reduced to "teeth" and arranged in whorls around the stem at the joint. Common on sandy, moist soil, in meadows, along roadside ditches, stream banks and railroad embankments.

Conditions of Poisoning

These plants contain, among other toxic principles, aconitic acid, equistitine, and thiaminase. Horses are much more susceptible to Equisetum than cattle.

Symptoms

Symptoms appear suddenly after the plant has been eaten, especially if the plant was in a dried condition. The first symptoms are unthriftiness, weakness, with loss of flesh. Appetite may or may not be affected. In a few weeks a lack of muscle control will be noticeable, and the animal will frequently fall. In advanced cases the symptoms are difficult breathing, pale mucous membranes, rapid and weak pulse, diarrhea, convulsion, coma, and then death.

Treatment

In early stages purgatives and stimulants should be given. The animal should be kept quiet, and high quality rations should be fed. Avoid feeding hay containing large quantities of the plant. Treatment with massive doses of thiamine seems to be effective except in advanced cases.

Description

Shoots similar, forming long, tapering canelike stalks, 1 to 6 feet high. Stems stiff, evergreen, with terminal spore-bearing cones. Leaves reduced to "teeth" and arranged in whorls around the stem at the joints. Common in wet localities, thickets, along streams, roadside ditches and borders of swamps, and in mountain sections of the state.

Coarse-growing perennial fern, with stout black horizontal rootstock. Frond or leaf broad, triangular in shape, and divided into three main parts, each of which is twice subdivided. Reproduction by spores borne in late summer on the lower edges of the mature fronds. Common in open acid woodlands and high pastures of the state.

Conditions of Poisoning

Not ordinarily eaten by stock, except during a dry season or in late summer when there is a scarcity of green herbage. Poisonous both fresh and dried in hay, though hogs eat the rootstocks without harm. The chemical action causing the poison is cumulative and symptoms often do not appear immediately. The toxic material is unknown.

Symptoms

Cattle affected usually have a high temperature, stand with head down and drool at the mouth. There is a rapid loss of flesh along with difficult breathing and excess salivation. Blood appears in the feces, either in bright red clots or as black feces. There is generally a trickle of blood from the nostrils, The mucous membranes will be congested, hemorrhagic or a yellow colour. These symptoms may be confused with anthrax.

In horses the first symptom noticed is an unsteady gait. Horses become drowsy, push their heads against solid objects and have difficulty swallowing. From 7 to 20 days after the symptoms are first noticed the animal will "go down." Death usually follows in several days.

Treatment

If the condition is diagnosed early enough, some animals will respond to treatment. Saline purgatives, raw linseed oil, mineral oil or melted lard should be given. Thiamine hydrochloride injected intravenously may be of some value.

Description

Evergreen shrub. Leaves alternate, needle-like, stiff, 1/2 to 1 inch long, dark green and glossy above and yellow-green on the lower surface. Seeds solitary, born in a cup-shaped, fleshy bright red fruit, appearing somewhat like a red berry.

Conditions of Poisoning

Poisonous properties have been attributed to the alkaloid, taxine, a heart depressant. The leaves, bark, wood and seeds are poisonous. When large amounts are eaten, death may result within a short time. Cattle, horses, sheep, goats, and wild animals have been poisoned by browsing the leaves and twigs. The red pulp of the fruits seems to be harmless, but seeds may contain the poisonous alkaloid. Poisoning sometimes occurs from livestock eating prunings and droppings. The red fruits are attractive to children.

Symptoms

Large doses usually result in sudden death without additional symptoms. Animals are found close to plants from which they have eaten, frequently with twigs or leaves still in their mouths. In subacute cases, typical symptoms include trembling, laboured breathing, and collapse. Spontaneous recovery in subacute cases has been reported, and, in such cases, the time between ingestion and evidence of symptoms may be as long as two days. Gastroenteritis and diarrhea may be evidenced in subacute cases.

Treatment

In acute cases, death occurs before any treatment can be administered. In less acute cases, atropine has been reported as an effective treatment to counteract the depressant effect of the alkaloid taxine.

Description

Large perennial, 3-6 feet high, with scaly, creeping rootstalks. Flowers in long, open, terminal panicle.

Sorghum: *Sorghum vulgare L.*

Description

Very sturdy annual. Tall, coarse grass with flowers similar to Johnson grass.

Sudan grass. *Sorghum vulgare var. sudanese (Piper) Hitch.*

Description

Annual, similar to sorghum, but of more slender growth. Neither sorghum nor sudan grass has scaly, creeping rootstalks.

All three are cultivated as forage crops, but Johnson grass is a weed of considerable importance in Kentucky, since it spreads rapidly into cultivated fields. Once established, it is hard to eradicate because of its underground rootstocks.

Conditions of Poisoning

Normally these grasses furnish excellent forage, and their use should not be discouraged. Since, under certain conditions, they may be dangerously poisonous, they should never be fed in a wilted or stunted condition to livestock. Cut hay and silage should be cured for at least six weeks before being used. These grasses should never be pastured until they are at least a foot tall; second growth is also very dangerous.

The toxic principle is hydrocyanic acid. Animals are more likely to be poisoned if they drink soon after eating plants of these species. Cattle are more susceptible than horses and sheep.

Symptoms

Lethal amounts of hydrocyanic acid cause respiratory paralysis and spasms, followed quickly by death. Animals are usually found dead before symptoms are noticed.

Smaller doses cause excitement and convulsions; later, depression sets in. Respirations are deep and accelerated at first but become weak and irregular. Pupils of the eyes are dilated and appear glassy. Nostrils and mouth are usually filled with foam. The animal may become bloated and urinate and defecate often. The breath will have an almond odour.

Treatment

If treatment is to be beneficial it should be started before respiratory paralysis begins to occur.

The best antidotes are either sodium nitrite, sodium thiosulfate or methylene blue, given intravenously. Calcium gluconate may also be helpful.

Conditions of Poisoning

Oaks seem to be most poisonous in the budding and leafing stages, which occur early in the spring when very little other forage is available. Animals turned into wooded areas before grass becomes abundant may consume large quantities of the buds and young leaves. Small amounts do not seem to be injurious, but when they are a large part of an animal's diet, severe illness can follow, often resulting in death of the animal two weeks to a month later. Cattle and sheep seem more susceptible to oak poisoning than other animals.

Tannic acid is considered to be the poisonous principle, although experimental feeding of tannic acid failed to produce the condition. Obviously, some other substance may be involved.

Symptoms

Constipation and loss of appetite are early symptoms. The feces are scanty, dry, and often contain mucus and blood. In some cases this may later be followed by profuse diarrhea. The affected animal usually exhibits a gaunt, tucked up appearance. There is evidence of jaundice, and blood or hemoglobin may appear in the urine. The muzzle may become dry and scaly. There is a reluctance on the part of the affected animal to follow the herd and a tendency to remain near water. When forced to move, severely affected animals show evidence of weakness and have a shuffling gait. They later collapse and die. Rarely are more than a few animals in a herd affected.

Treatment

Animals grazing wooded areas in the spring should be watched for early evidence of oak poisoning. If it occurs, animals should be moved to other pastures. In early or mild cases of oak poisoning, veterinarians may administer symptomatic treatment with good success. However, for severely poisoned animals no effective treatment is known.

Other common names are snowdrop and nap-at-noon. Star-of-Bethlehem is becoming more common as a lawn weed in Kentucky. It was introduced from Europe, and some people still consider it an ornamental plant. Where star-of-Bethlehem is a weed problem, the plants have escaped from cultivation, and in many cases almost completely crowd out desirable lawn grasses.

Description

Star-of-Bethlehem is a perennial that reproduces mostly by bulbs, rarely by seed. It belongs to the same family as wild garlic (lily family) and may be confused with wild garlic. Star-of-Bethlehem does not, however, have the strong scent of onion or garlic, and the leaves are about as long as the stem and have a light green midrib. The stems develop from small bulbs that are usually in clumps, grow to a height of from 4 to 12 inches, and bear several white star-shaped flowers.

In Kentucky, new growth starts in late January or early February. The plant grows to maturity and develops flowers in May or early June. The tops then die, leaving brown areas in the lawn throughout the summer.

Conditions of Poisoning

All parts of the plant are poisonous when eaten either fresh or in hay. It is reported to contain uncharacterised alkaloids. The bulb seems to be more toxic than other parts of the plant.

Description

Tall, smooth, perennial herb with a large taproot. Stems succulent, purplish, 3 to 10 feet high. Leaves alternate, pointed, narrowly oblong, with smooth margins. Flowers small, white, borne in long, drooping clusters. Fruits flattened, spherical, dark purple berries, usually with ten seeds. Common on recently cleared land, in open woods, pastures, and along fence rows.

Conditions of Poisoning

A saponin-like substance, in addition to the alkaloid, phytolaccine, is present in all parts of the plant, especially the roots and seeds. Cooking destroys the poison and young shoots are sometimes used as cooked greens. Although animals usually avoid pokeweed due to its unpleasant taste, early in the spring they sometimes feed on the young shoots. Cases have been reported of poisoning in pigs from rooting out and consuming the roots of the plant. It has also been reported that in Kentucky cattle were attracted to pokeweed plant treated with certain herbicides, thus causing loss of several animals.

Symptoms

In most cases when small amounts are eaten, the only symptoms are retching and vomiting, usually noticed several hours after the plant has been eaten. If larger amounts are eaten, spasms, diarrhea, and convulsions will be the main symptoms. The cause of death is respiratory paralysis.

Treatment

Tannic acid, mineral oil and stimulants will help in most cases if the condition is diagnosed early enough

Description

Stout perennial, 4-35 inches high. Leaves alternate and very deeply lobed. Flowers spurred, blue or occasionally white, arranged in terminal clusters, appearing in spring. The root is a tuberous cluster.

Commonly found in rich, open woods and along streams.

The annual larkspur (Delphinium Ajacis L.), which often escapes from gardens and establishes itself as a weed in fields and roadsides, is also poisonous.

Conditions of Poisoning

Larkspur contains several very poisonous alkaloids, including delphinine, and is most poisonous in the early stages of growth, during April and May. Poisoning occurs when stock grazes in woodland pastures before other green herbage is available. Cattle are the most susceptible, but horses and sheep can be poisoned by eating large quantities.

Symptoms

The symptoms of larkspur poisoning differ according to the amount eaten and the animal's tolerance. Small amounts may cause loss of appetite; excitability, staggering, and constipation. Severe symptoms that develop when an animal eats large quantities are slobbering, vomiting, colic, bloating, and convulsions. Death is due to respiratory paralysis.

Treatment

Protect animals from excitement by keeping them in a quiet place and give them such drugs as chloral hydrate or one of the barbiturates. Epsom salts may be given to help the constipation. Other drugs should be given to relieve the animal. It may be necessary to treat the animal for bloat. Dutchman's breeches, staggerweed, wild bleeding heart. Dicentra Cucullaria L. Bernh.

Description

Delicate perennial with finely cut fern-like leaves. Small yellow pea-like tubers arranged along the underground stem. Flowers 1 to 10, creamy white with 2 short rounded projections, and arranged on slender stalks.

Description

Closely resembles squirrel corn but small grain-like tubers are clustered at the base of the stem. Flowers with 2 spur-like projections. Both species are among the earliest of spring plants, blossoming in April or May. Common in rich open woods, often in company with dwarf larkspur.

Conditions of Poisoning

The entire plants of both species contain a number of poisonous alkaloids. Dutchman's breeches is more poisonous than squirrel corn. These plants are unpalatable and are not frequently eaten in harmful quantities when other forage is available. Most cases of poisoning occur in early spring (April or May) when animals are grazing in wooded areas. Cows are more frequently poisoned than horses; sheep are not affected.

Symptoms

A staggering gait and a loss of milk production. Later symptoms are sudden trembling which increases in severity, frothing of the mouth, laboured breathing, diarrhea and convulsions. Most animals will recover, if the dosage is not too heavy, and if they are kept away from the plants after the first symptoms appear.

Treatment

Animals showing "staggers" in the spring should be moved to clean pastures at once. If poisoning symptoms are severe, purgatives, mineral oil and stimulants may be given.

Description

Tree or shrub with slender horizontal branches. Bark of young branches and twigs reddish-brown with prominent white lenticels (pores). Leaves alternate, simple, elliptical, pointed, margins finely toothed, leathery in texture, and usually have a row of hairs on the lower surface along both sides of the midrib. Flowers small, white, in drooping clusters, and produce dark-red to black cherry fruits.

Common along fence rows, roadside thickets, and in rich, open woods. Choke-cherry (Prunus virginiana L.), also poisonous, is of limited distribution in Kentucky.

Conditions of Poisoning

Wild cherries contain the glucoside amygdalin, which, by a series of chemical changes, is converted to hydrocyanic acid. This acid is formed very rapidly in wilted or bruised leaves, particularly those on young tender shoots. Most cases of poisoning occur when animals have access to wilted leaves on branches blown down during wind or hail storms, or branches that have been clipped or pruned.

Symptoms

Symptoms may develop very rapidly after an animal has eaten wilted wild cherry leaves. The poisoned animal becomes uneasy, staggers, and has convulsions. Breathing will be very difficult and the mucous membranes become blue. Death may come so quickly that the animal will be found near the wilted leaves or tree.

Treatment

If the condition is diagnosed in time, intravenous injection of sodium thiosulfate and sodium nitrite will save the animal. Calcium dextrose may be helpful. In most cases the animal will be dead before a veterinarian can be called.

Description

Moderate-sized tree, often with 2 short spines at base of leafs talk, bark rough. Leaves alternate, pinnately compound; the individual leaflets oval-shaped, without teeth. Flowers creamy white, fragrant, sweet-pea like, arranged in long, drooping clusters. Fruit a flat, brown pod, 1/2 inch wide, 2 to 4 inches long, and containing 4-8 small kidney-shaped beans.. Common in woods and thickets. Often planted as an ornamental and for erosion control, but has spread widely as a "weed" tree along highways and in waste places.

Conditions of Poisoning

The poisonous substance is a phytotoxin, robin. Animals are affected by eating the young shoots, leaves, pods, seeds, and by gnawing on the bark, or drinking water in which the pods have been soaked. All farm animals are susceptible.

Symptoms

Animals will become stupid, not notice their surroundings, and stand with the legs apart. Heart action is irregular and breathing is feeble, mucous membranes are yellow, and the pupil of the eye dilated. Colic pains may be present and soon followed by diarrhea. Cattle are quite often dizzy and very nervous.

Treatment

Death follows the onset of symptoms unless treatment is started soon. An injection of digitalis to help the heart action is useful. Other treatments used are just to help decrease the symptoms and give ease to the animal.

Description

Tree or shrub. Leaves opposite, palmately compound (leaflets arranged like the fingers of a hand). Leaflets usually five. Flowers yellowish, in large clusters at ends of branches. Fruit a prickly capsule (at least when young), leathery, 1 to 3 seeded-each seed glossy brown with a pale scar-hence the common name buckeye. Bark with a strong, offensive odour. Common in rich, moist woods, and along river banks.

Similar to Ohio buckeye, but leaflets usually seven and flowers white. A cultivated species introduced from Europe and widely planted as an ornamental shade tree.

Similar to Ohio buckeye, but bark with a slight odour, and fruits not prickly. Common in rich, moist woods and along river banks.

Conditions of Poisoning

These plants contain poisonous alkaloids and glucosides, especially in the young shoots, nuts, and sprouts. Poisoning is most likely to occur in early spring in woodland pastures where there are sprouts and seedlings.

Symptoms

Buckeye poisoning affects the central nervous system, causing an uneasy, staggering gait. The animal will be weak, have severe trembling, and may vomit. Mucous membranes will be congested and the pupils of the eye will be dilated. The animal then will go into a coma before death.

Treatment

Quite often the animal is found dead before any treatment can be given. If cases are found soon enough, stimulants and purgatives are indicated.

Description

Erect, freely branching perennial, 1 to 3 feet tall. Leaves opposite, less than 1/2 inch wide, oblong or linear in shape, with smooth margins, and covered with transparent dots. Many yellow flowers in somewhat flattened clusters at the top of the, stem. Petals with black, glandular dots on the margins. The fruit is a three-parted capsule containing many small, dark-brown seeds.

Abundant in old meadows, pastures, wastelands, and along the roadside.

Conditions of Poisoning

The poisonous action of this plant is probably due to two fluorescent substances, hypericin and hypericum red. When white-skinned animals feed on large quantities of St. Johnswort in the flowering stage, their skins may become extremely sensitive to sunlight, a condition called photosensitisation. Dark-skinned animals have enough pigment to screen out the undesirable light rays.

Other plants that may cause similar symptoms are alsike clover and buckwheat.

Symptoms

White-skinned animals, animals with white spots or belts, or sheep that have been sheared, quite often develop a dermatitis, the result of light sensitisation. The most typical symptoms are skin blisters, falling hair and scabs. The skin may become dry and crack open. Poisoning is rarely fatal. In some cases in sheep, paralysis has been noted.

Treatment

Remove animals from the pasture as soon as possible and put them in a cool, dark barn. Apply oil to the affected areas. Supply plenty of fresh water and feed.

Description

Smooth biennial herb, 3 to 8 feet high, with purple-spotted stem and finely-divided compound leaves. Flowers small, white, in umbels, blossom in early summer. Leaves have a rank, disagreeable odour. Poison hemlock can be distinguished from 'Water hemlock by more finely-divided leaves and a long, parsnip-like root. Extremely common along roadsides, banks of streams, ditches, in fields, and around farm buildings.

Conditions of Poisoning

Poisoning is most likely to occur in early spring when leaves are green and other pasturage is not available. The entire plant is poisonous. Cases of human poisoning have occurred from mistakenly eating the seeds, leaves, and roots for anise, parsley or parsnips. The toxic principle is the volatile alkaloid, coniine. Although drying reduces the coniine content, hay containing the dried plants is not entirely safe.

Symptoms

Poisoning generally appears suddenly, and the owner finds the animal "down." Some of the symptoms that may be noticed are: excessive salivation (slobbering), loss of appetite, muscular weakness or twitching of the muscles, incoordination, rapid pulse and great pain. Death occurs from respiratory paralysis.

Treatment

If animals are found and diagnosed early enough, purgatives may be given to empty the digestive tract. Intestinal astringents such as tannic acid are useful. Nerve and heart stimulants may be given.

Description

Evergreen shrub, 3-9 feet high. Leaves to five inches long, alternate or irregular, leathery, shiny, light green on lower surface. Flowers pink or white, cup-shaped, borne in spring. Common in upland woods, hilly pastures, and on acid soil.

Evergreen shrub or small tree. Leaves alternate, leathery, whitish or rusty on lower surfaces. Flowers bell-shaped, rose-pink to white. Common in damp woods, swamps, and upland areas.

Conditions of Poisoning

Mountain laurel and rhododendron contain a resinous substance, andromedotoxin. Sheep are more frequently poisoned than other livestock, since they are often pastured in areas that are better adapted for the growth of these plants.

Symptoms

In certain sections of the state, quite a few animals are lost each year from eating laurel and rhododendron. If an animal eats 0.2% of its body weight, symptoms may develop. The first symptom is irregular breathing. Later, slobbering at the mouth, grating of the teeth, vomiting, staggering, blindness, stupor, and then death. The meat from these animals should not be eaten. If the animal recovers, several days should elapse before it is used for human consumption.

Treatment

If the animals are found early enough, oil drenches, with materials such as mineral oil, raw linseed oil, lard, etc. should be given.

Description

Branching perennial, 1 1/2 to 5 feet high. Stem contains a milky juice or latex and arises from a vertical underground rootstock. Leaves opposite, oblong in shape, with smooth margins. Flowers greenish-white, borne in clusters at the ends of the stems and branches. Fruit a long, slender pod containing many seeds that bear tufts of "floss."

Common in gravelly soil, along roadsides, in fields, meadows and wastelands, often in large colonies.

Conditions of Poisoning

Indian hemp contains the glucoside cymarin, poisonous resins and possibly other toxic substances. All parts of the plant are poisonous, either fresh or dried in hay. As little as 1/2 to 1 ounce of the fresh green leaves can cause death to a cow.

Symptoms

A rise in body temperature, sweating, strong pulse, ears and legs become cold, pupils of the eyes usually dilated, and the inside of the mouth becomes red and sore. Bowel action is frequent. In advanced cases death will usually occur.

Treatment

If cases are diagnosed early enough, the stomach should be emptied and gallic or tannic acid given as an antidote. Heart stimulants are sometimes helpful. Keep the animal in a quiet place and give it good feed and water.

Description

Stems solitary or clustered, 1-5 feet high. Leaves opposite. Flowers pink to rose-purple, arranged in umbels. Fruit a pod containing seeds tufted with "floss."

Description

Erect perennial, 2-4 feet high, stem with broad opposite or whorled leaves and milky sap. Flowers dull pink, arranged in simple umbels. Fruit a pod containing seeds tufted with "floss."

Description

Erect perennial 1-3 feet high, stems with alternate leaves and no milky sap. Flowers bright orange, arranged in simple umbels. Fruit a pod containing seeds tufted with "floss."

Description

Slender perennial, 1-3 feet high. Leaves arranged in whorls, very narrow with curled margins. Flowers greenish-white, in small umbels. Fruit a pod containing seeds tufted with "floss."

Conditions of Poisoning

A resinous substance is located in the stems and leaves. The plants are poisonous both fresh and dried. Green plants are rarely eaten because of their bitter, acrid taste. Whorled milkweed is more poisonous than the broad-leaved species. Milkweeds of the western plains of the United States are among the most deadly of the poisonous plants.

Symptoms

The first symptoms are loss of appetite and diarrhea. Later, the animal will stagger, fall and develop paralysis of the rear limbs. Breathing will be laboured and spasms violent. Death is due to respiratory failure. Autopsies show congestion of liver, kidneys, heart, lungs and nervous system.

Treatment

Sedatives, such as chloral hydrate and the barbiturates are helpful in easing the pain. Mineral oil will be helpful in early stages.

Description

A stout, coarse annual, 2 to 5 feet tall, with spreading branches. Leaves alternate, coarsely toothed, green or purplish and strongly scented. Flowers trumpet shaped, large, white or purplish. Fruit a hard, spiny capsule that splits into 4 valves at maturity.

Common in cultivated fields and waste places, often abundant in barnyards and abandoned pastures.

Conditions of Poisoning

Jimson weed contains the poisonous alkaloids, hyoscyamine and hyoscine. The entire plant is poisonous, both green and dried. Because of its strong odour and bitter taste, the green plant is rarely eaten. Humans may be poisoned by eating the fruits.

Symptoms

Common symptoms in cattle are rapid pulse and respiration, dry mouth and, possibly, a complete retention of urine, or frequent urination. Diarrhea, dilation of the pupils of the eyes, and stiffness may occur. Close to death, the respirations become slow, irregular, and weak. Death is caused by asphyxia, Quite often this weed grows in the hog lot and may be the cause of some deaths. The main symptom in hogs is convulsive twitching of the entire body.

Treatment

If animals are found early enough, mineral oil is helpful, since it acts as a purge and coats the walls of the intestines. Tannic acid is used to precipitate the alkaloids. Stimulants and molasses are helpful.

Description

Low, branched annual, 1 to 2 feet high, with angular stems. Leaves alternate, oval, thin textured, with wavy margins. Flowers white, in drooping clusters on lateral stalks between the leaves, somewhat resembling tomato flowers. Fruit a berry, green when immature, turning purplish-black at maturity. A common weed in open woods, fields, waste places, and around farm buildings.

Conditions of Poisoning

The alkaloidal glucoside, solanine, is present in the leaves, stems and green berries. The plants are less toxic when dried. Most cases of poisoning occur among sheep, goats, calves, pigs and poultry, as mature horses and cows rarely eat enough to be seriously affected.

Symptoms

The first symptoms are weakness, stupor, staggering gait and constipation, followed by dilated pupils, loss of muscular coordination and sense of feeling. In more advanced cases, cramps and convulsions are typical. The animal will soon die of respiratory paralysis. The progress of the symptoms is often rapid.

Treatment

There is no treatment for nightshade poisoning. Sedatives will help stop the convulsions.

Description

Hairy annual with leafy branched stem, 1 to 2 feet high. Leaves thin, oval or oblong, with toothed margins. Flowers two-lipped, pale-blue, inconspicuous, borne in the axils of the upper leaves. Fruit a capsule covered by the swollen inflated calyx. Common in meadows, pastures and cultivated fields.

Perennial herb to a height of 3 feet. Stem leafy, rather stout, and usually unbranched. Flowers about 3/4 inch long, deep blue, in a dense terminal spike.

Commonly found in roadside ditches, swampy areas, wet pastures, and along the edge of streams and ponds.

Conditions of Poisoning

Poisonous alkaloids and volatile oils are present in the leaves, stems and fruits. In heavily infested pastures or during dry seasons, when other green forage is scarce, animals occasionally eat the plants in sufficient quantities to be seriously poisoned.

Symptoms

Nausea, vomiting and dilated pupils. The animal will stagger, get down, have convulsions, go into a coma and then die.

Treatment

Gallic or tannic acid is the best treatment, along with stimulants. Mineral oil is helpful in lining the digestive system.

Description

A smooth, erect, perennial herb, 1 to 5 feet high. Leaves opposite, oval, with pointed tips and sharply-toothed edges, strongly resembling the leaves of nettles. The upper surface of the leaf dull, and the lower shiny. Each leaf has 3 prominent main veins on the underside. In late summer the small white flowers appear in compound clusters. Found in woods; damp, shady pastures; and, occasionally, thickets and clearings.

Conditions of Poisoning

Tremetol, a poisonous alcohol, is present in the leaves and stems. This toxic principle may be transmitted through the milk of poisoned cows to humans, causing the disease known as "milk sickness" or "trembles." Animals are usually poisoned during the late summer when forage is scarce. The effect is cumulative. Animals may die from eating a large amount of the plant at one time, or from eating small amounts over a long period of time.

Symptoms

Cows appear listless, have severe constipation, violent trembling, and their breath will become foul with a peculiar acetone odour. Joints become stiff, the animal falls and refuses to rise or otherwise exert itself, grinds its teeth, has rapid, laboured breathing, and may die.

In horses, the first stage is general sluggishness, marked depression, and slight incoordination of the muscles, especially of the hind parts. The trembling stage, so characteristic of poisoned cattle, is sometimes absent. An inability to swallow, due to paralysis of the throat muscles, accompanied by a nasal discharge, will show up as the disease progresses.

Human symptoms include severe constipation, vomiting, foul breath, subnormal temperature, weakness, delirium and collapse.

Treatment

Since poisoning usually occurs in late summer, cattle should be removed about the first of July from areas infested with this weed.

When the animal reaches the trembling stage, there is little you can do. Strong purgatives will help eliminate the drug from the digestive tract. Stimulants and calcium gluconate are helpful. Keep the cow milked out to eliminate the poison, but do not use the milk for human consumption.

Description

Erect-growing coarse perennial, 2 to 6 feet tall, with narrowly-winged stem. Leaves alternate, lance-shaped and coarsely toothed. Flowers yellow, resembling small sunflowers. Toothed ray flowers are characteristically turned downwards. Another species, the purple-headed sneezeweed (Helenium nudiflorum Nutt:) is less present in the state.

Commonly found around water holes, streams and ditches, and in swampy pastures and meadows.

Description

Annual, 1-2 feet high, with fine, narrow leaves. Flowers similar to sneezeweed.

Usually found in fields, pastures, cultivated areas, and around farm buildings. Extremely common in western Kentucky.

Conditions of Poisoning

Most cases of serious poisoning occur in the late summer and early fall when the plants come into bloom. Sheep, cattle and horses are susceptible. Most livestock avoid these plants, but individual animals may eat sufficient quantities to cause death. The plants are poisonous either fresh or cured in hay. Cows grazing on these plants may produce milk with a bitter flavor.

Symptoms

Rapid pulse, restlessness, difficult breathing, and loss of muscular control followed by plunging and staggering blindly. At this time the animals are extremely sensitive to the touch. After eating large quantities of the blossoms, the animals may die suddenly with spasms and convulsions.

Treatment

If the milk is bitter or the animal is showing symptoms of poisoning, remove all the stock to clean, weed-free pastures. Melted lard or mineral oil is helpful if given early enough.

Description

Branching annual, 1 to 3 feet high. Stems angled, sometimes red-spotted. Leaves alternate, hairy, rough in texture, somewhat heart-shaped, and variously toothed and lobed. Flowers inconspicuous, of two kinds-those in terminal spikes produce only pollen, while those in clusters in the axils of the leaves produce the seed. Fruit a hard, oval, prickly bur, about 3/4 inch long, containing two seeds.

The seedlings have small strap-shaped leaves, 1/4 inch wide and 11/4 inches long, and later produce the more characteristic leaves. They sprout from the buried burs. Several species of cocklebur are common in Kentucky. They differ in the shape and hairiness of the bur, but all are poisonous in the seedling stage.

Common in waste places, cultivated fields, along roadsides, beds of dry ponds, and on overflowed lands along streams.

Conditions of Poisoning

The poisonous substance is a glucoside, xanthostrumarin, found in germinating seeds and young seedlings. Since the toxicity decreases as the plants develop, the mature plant is probably non-poisonous. Hogs are most frequently poisoned, but cattle and sheep are also susceptible. Mature plants are seldom eaten, but the ripe spiny burs may result in purely mechanical injury.

Symptoms

Depression, often accompanied by nausea and, occasionally, vomiting. The affected animal becomes gaunt, weak, and unable to stand, has laboured respiration and a rapid, weak pulse. It may lie on its side and move its legs in a running fashion until completely exhausted.

Within 24 hours after eating 0.75% of its own weight of young seedling plants, the animal may show signs of poisoning, and even die. If death does not occur, several weeks will pass before the animal is back to normal.

Treatment

Give emergency treatment with fatty substances, such as mineral oil, cream or even whole milk, by mouth or through a stomach tube.

Description

A large tree with rough bark, ranging from 60 to 80 feet in height. The trunk, which is relatively short and 1 to 2 feet in diametre, divides into numerous large branches that end in contorted, stout twigs. The leaf is twice pinnately compound, being made up of a hundred or more separate oval leaflets arranged on branches of the rib. Its fruit is a flat, leathery pod, 4 to 6 inches in length, containing 4 to 7 hard, flat, dark brown seeds. Pods often remain on the tree until late winter. The tree usually grows on rich bottom land and along streams, scattered among other trees.

Conditions of Poisoning

Poisoning is apt to occur in late winter or early spring when other forage is scarce and animals eat quantities of the pods and seeds lying on the ground, or nibble on young shoots. Cases of poisoning from Kentucky coffee tree are not common, but they may be fatal. The poisonous principle is said to be an alkaloid known as cytisin which is found in the leaves, pods, and seeds.

Symptoms

These have not been well described, although, in reported cases, animals seemed to show evidence of severe pain shortly after feeding on leaves and pods. Profuse diarrhea with straining has also been reported. At autopsy of these animals, a white, sticky mucus was present in the small intestine with congestion of the mucous membranes, and foamy fecal matter was found in the large intestine.

Treatment

There is no specific or reliable treatment. Veterinarians may give symptomatic treatments that have proved valuable in other plant alkaloid poisonings. However, recovery will depend largely on severity of the poisoning.

Supplementary List of Poisonous Plants

Many of the species listed below are of limited abundance and distribution in Kentucky. Others are so distasteful that they are rarely eaten, while still others contain so little toxic substance that very large amounts are necessary to cause serious poisoning. A few cultivated species are included. Although generally less troublesome than the plants previously discussed, the species listed here should not be overlooked when confusing cases of poisoning are encountered.

Ergot (Claviceps Purpurea (Fr.) Tul.)

Ergot is a fungus or mold that grows in the flower heads of various grasses, perhaps most frequently on rye and redtop. It produces a hard black kernel in the place of the seed. Animals may be poisoned by eating ergot-infected grain or by grazing on infected grass. The poisoning may be acute if large quantities of ergot are eaten at one time, or the results may be slow and cumulative if small amounts are eaten regularly. Symptoms include abortion in pregnant animals, gangrenous conditions, muscular trembling and incoordination, dullness and depression. The ergot (Claviceps paspali S. and H.) that occurs on Dallis grass and other native species of Paspalum is also poisonous, causing characteristic nervousness and trembling.

Jack-in-the-pulpit, Indian turnip (Arisaema atrorubens (Ait.) Blume)

Plants of this species are more common in the mountain and wooded sections of the state. Poisoning may occur from eating large amounts of the fresh leaves and corms. Animals usually avoid them because of their bitter, acrid taste. Symptoms are those of intestinal inflammation and colic. Burning sensations in the mouth and throat will cause the animals to drink constantly.

Hemp, Marijuana (Cannabis sativa L.)

A weed around fields where it was formerly cultivated as a crop. Hemp is not ordinarily eaten by animals, but may be consumed in sufficient quantity to cause narcotic poisoning.

Buttercup (Ranunculus spp.) All animals may be poisoned by eating the fresh plants. Moonseed (Menisperum canadense L.) A climbing vine, with small clusters of grape-like fruits that are poisonous to humans. White sweet clover (Melilotus alba Desr.) Yellow sweet clover (Melilotus officinalis L. Lam) Sweet clovers are valuable forage crops and can be used freely as pasture, but poisoning may occur when livestock are fed exclusively on spoiled sweet clover hay or silage. Poisoned animals show symptoms of hemorrhage with marked swellings on various parts of the body, and may bleed to death at calving time or from such minor operations as castration or dehorning. Treatment consists of transfusions of normal blood to restore the blood clotting powers.

Alsike Clover (Trifolium hybridum L.)

Animals should not be grazed on this clover when it is wet or dew-covered. Under certain conditions alsike clover may affect white-skinned animals by making them light sensitive.

Spurges (Euphorbia spp.)

Livestock may exhibit symptoms of digestive irritations and weakness if fed for an extended period of time on hay containing spurges. Severe blistering of the skin may result from contact with the milky sap.

Castor Bean, Castor Oil Plant (Ricinus communis L.)

Commonly grown as an ornamental, this plant often persists as a weed in fields and along roadsides. All parts of the plant are poisonous. Symptoms are nausea, vomiting, thirst, dullness of vision, and convulsions. Severe cases of poisoning may result from eating large quantities, and may cause death.

Hogwort, Wooly Croton (Croton capitatus Michx.)

Animals are sometimes affected from eating hogwort with hay. Symptoms are diarrhea, colic and general nervousness.

Boxwood (Buxus sempervirens L.)

Although grown extensively as an ornamental hedge, clippings and branches may produce fatal results if eaten.

Climbing Bittersweet (Celastrus scandens L.)

A woody vine with attractive clusters of red and orange berries. Leaves and fruits are poisonous. Bittersweet acts both as a heart poison and purgative, producing nausea and prostration.

Ground ivy, Gill-over-the-ground, Creeping Charlie (Glechoma hederacea L.)

Common in lawns, neglected fields and fence rows. Mildly poisonous if large quantities are eaten fresh or dried in hay.

Blue Nightshade, European Nightshade (Solanum dulcamara L.)

Resembles black nightshade, previously discussed, except that the leaves are lobed at the base and the berry is red instead of black when mature. The leaves and fruits are toxic.

Horse Nettle, Bull Nettle (Solanum carolinense L.)

Prickly coarse-stemmed perennial, 8 inches to 2 feet high. Common in pastures and cultivated fields. Animals ordinarily do not eat these weeds unless harvested in hay. Chronic poisoning with symptoms of general unthriftiness may result from prolonged eating of small quantities. If a considerable quantity is eaten within a few hours, digestive disturbances, sleepiness and paralysis may occur.

Tobacco (Nicotiana Tabacum L.)

Although usually not eaten by livestock, a few cases of poisoning have been reported.

Matrimony Vine (Lycium halimifolium Mill.)

Frequently escapes from cultivation. Leaves and young shoots may be poisonous.

Buttonbush (Cephalanthus occidentalis L.)

A shrub, found in moist, swampy areas. The fruits resemble the buttonballs of the sycamore tree. Most poisoning occurs when animals have eaten the leaves.

Elderberry, Black Eider (Sambucus canadensis L.)

Common shrub in fields, along fence rows and at the edge of woods. Leaves opposite, pinnately compound. Numerous small white flowers in large clusters develop into purple-black berries. Most cases of poisoning occur when animals eat, the new growth in the spring. Symptoms and treatment are similar to those for wild black cherry. Small herbaceous plants, in wet swampy meadows and pastures, producing yellow, daisy-like flowers in early spring. Plants consumed in large quantities, either fresh or in hay, may affect livestock.

Plants Causing Mechanical Injury

Numerous plants that are common in Kentucky but not poisonous possess sharp awns, burs, or spines which may cause mechanical injury to animals. Examples are the tearing of the flesh around the eyes and mouth; crippling, resulting from getting into hooves; or ulcerous conditions or hair balls in the digestive tract. A few of the most common plants in this category are: barley and wild barley (Hordeum spp.), burdock (Arctium minus), downy brome-grass (Bromus tectorum), foxtails (Setaria spp.), Russian thistle (Salsola Kali L. var. tenuifolia Meyer), sandbur (Cenchrus pauciflorus), spring amaranth (Amaranthus spinosus) and thistle (Cirsium vulgare).

Azalea Toxicity in Goats

Azaleas can be toxic to goats, and even a small amount of the plant's foliage can result in poisoning. The poisoning may be from an animal "brows-ing" among the azaleas (*Rhododendron indica*). Or occasionally, poisoning occurs due to well-meaning individuals throwing azalea clippings to nearby goats. Azaleas are found worldwide and have been responsible for numerous instances of poisoning in livestock, humans and pets. These evergreen, semi-evergreen, or deciduous shrubs with flowers of various colours are frequently found as ornamentals in the southeastern United States. For goats, fresh foliage at 0.1 percent of the goat's body weight may be toxic (That means 0.1 pound or 1.6 ounces of fresh azalea foliage could be toxic to a 100 pound goat). Nectar and honey made from the flowers of these plants may also be toxic. Ingestion of toxic amounts of the azalea plant often results in development of the following clinical signs within six hours of exposure:

- Depression and head pressing
- Severe salivation
- Abdominal cramps and bloat
- Vomiting/regurgitation
- Muscle tremors.

In severe cases, animals may develop an abnormal cardiac rhythm, hypotension (low blood pressure) convulsions and high fever (up to 106 degrees° F). Occasionally, affected animals vomit and then inhale part of what they are thowing up, causing a severe pneumonia which may result in death. Diagnosis usually is made on the basis of a history of exposure and display of typical clinical signs. Finding plant parts in what an animal has regurgitated can also be used to confirm the diagnosis. Recently, how-ever, tests have been developed to detect the toxin, grayano toxin, in the feces and/or urine of animals suspected of having consumed azaleas. This test can be used as a diagnostic tool when history is unavailable or clinical signs are deceptive.

There is no specific treatment for azalea toxicity. Supportive care, including administration of intravenous fluids, may be recommended by your veterinarian. Although animals can recover if treated promptly, azalea poisoning often is fatal for goats. Owners should make every effort to prevent exposure of goats to azaleas through such means as securely fencing them away from the plants. Goats seem to be attracted to the taste of azaleas and will readily consume them.

Poisoning of Livestock by Plants

There are many plants which contain chemicals or which accumulate chemicals that are poisonous to livestock. The results of poisoning can range from minor irritations and slightly lowered animal performance to severe cases where the animal is in a great deal of distress and may die. This Factsheet is an introduction to the ways and means that plants can poison livestock. It also describes plants which mechanically injure animals or may cause irritation of skin on contact. For additional information on weeds that are poisonous.

It would simplify matters if plants could be classified into two groups, poisonous and non-poisonous. Unfortunately, this cannot be done for many factors are responsible for the toxic principles in plants. What may be a harmless plant species in one circumstance could be deadly in another.

There are many plant factors that contribute to the toxic principles in plants. Individual plant species and varieties may differ in their poisonous content from early growth to maturity. With some plants, there is an increase in their ability to poison with advanced stages of growth, whereas with others the danger lessens. The state of the plant when eaten may also be important. In some cases, damage to the plant or wilting may produce poisonous chemicals in the plant which were not present in the fresh material. In other cases, such as with buttercups, the poison is contained in the fresh plants but not dried ones. Certain parts of a plant may be poisonous and other parts not. Rhubarb is a good example. The leaf stalk is eatable while the leaves are very poisonous.

Animal factors also influence the ability of plants to poison. Different animal species are susceptible to different plants and poisons. The age of the animal is also important. Young animals are often more susceptible than older ones, but it isn't always the case. Animals may build up resistance to certain poisons by being exposed to small quantities at first.

Then, if a large quantity is consumed, they are resistant because their metabolism has already adjusted to handle the poison. An animal that is hungry or has certain dietary deficiencies is more likely to eat toxic quantities of a poisonous plant than a well fed animal.

Classification of Poisons

There is a large variety of toxic substances that have been associated with plant poisonings. Unfortunately for many plant species, the nature of the toxic substance has not yet been identified. However, most of the important poisonous plants in Ontario contain toxic agents from one or more of the following groups.

Alkaloids

Alkaloids are organic basic substances with a bitter taste, examples of which are morphine, atropine, nicotine, quinine and strychnine. The alkaloids generally are irritating to the gastrointestinal tract producing nausea, colic and diarrhea and also act on the central nervous system to produce blindness, muscular weakness, convulsions and death. Toxic alkaloids are found in the following plants; swamp and death camas, lupines, buttercups, marshmarigolds, larkspur, the nightshades, squirrel corn and Dutchman's breeches.

Glycosides

Glycosides are natural plant products that contain the sugar glucose. They can be subdivided into three main groups.

Cyanogenic Glycosides

Cyanogenic glycosides are not themselves poisonous but in the presence of certain enzymes are hydrolyzed and produce hydrocyanic acid (HCN) which is highly toxic. HCN interferes with the oxygen exchange from the lungs to the body tissues so that various tissues including the brain are starved for oxygen and are consequently injured. The symptoms are muscle tremors, difficult, rapid respiration and convulsions. Often these are not seen because death occurs within minutes.

There are many factors that influence the amount of cyanogenic glycosides in plants. Some plant species normally have high levels, the highest levels occurring in early growth stages and decreasing as the plants mature. Climatic conditions, soil factors, shade and other factors that slow plant growth and development increase cyanogenic glycoside content. Low soil moisture, high nitrogen and low phosphorus all favour HCN production. Wilting, frost and other forms of physical damage to plants may induce a rapid increase in HCN content.

Cyanogenic glycosides occur in sorghums, sudan grass, marsh-arrow grass and wild cherries.

Saponin Glycosides

Saponin glycosides produce a violent gastroenteritis with vomiting, diarrhea and colic. If the saponin glycosides are absorbed into the bloodstream, they cause a breakdown of red blood cells and injury to the central nervous system producing convulsions and paralysis. This form of glycoside is found in purple cockle, cow cockle, bouncingbet and pokeweed.

Mustard Oil Glucosides

Mustard oil glucosides found in plants belonging to the Mustard family cause severe gastroenteritis. Symptoms are severe colic and purging.

Nitrate

Nitrate poisoning of animals is actually nitrite poisoning occurring when nitrate is reduced to nitrite in the gastrointestinal tract. The nitrite is absorbed into the bloodstream where it reacts with hemoglobin to form methemoglobin. This compound, which is brown in colour, is incapable of releasing oxygen. In acute cases of poisoning in cattle, 60 to 80% of the total hemoglobin is comprised of methemoglobin. Sheep generally do not develop as much methemoglobin and are therefore more resistant to this form of poisoning.

The symptoms of acute poisoning are trembling, staggering, rapid breathing, and death. Chronic poisoning may result in poor growth, poor milk production and abortions. In cattle, there is evidence that vitamin A storage is affected.

Some plant species are naturally good accumulators of nitrates. Common plant species that are associated with nitrate poisoning are shown in Table 1. The legume and grass species that are used for pastures or hay crops are not considered good nitrate accumulators, but given the right conditions can accumulate concentrations of nitrate that are potentially hazardous.

There is a direct response in plant nitrate concentration to increasing levels of nitrogen fertilization. Nitrate accumulation is greater when nitrate fertilizers are used than when either urea or ammonium sulfate is the nitrogen source.

A number of environmental conditions can influence the accumulation of nitrates in plants by altering mineral metabolism in the plant. Drought, uneven distribution of rainfall, and low light intensity have each been identified as climatic factors that bring about an accumulation of nitrates and nitrites in the stems and leaves of plants.

Molybdenum

Molybdenum poisoning can occur when there are abnormally high quantities of molybdenum in the soil. Animals pasturing on areas that meet this condition are often subject to acute scouring. The animals become emaciated, produce less milk, and their coats become rough and often faded. Legumes, particularly red and alsike clovers, are usually associated with molybdenum poisoning. To counteract the effect of molybdenum, it is necessary to add copper to the diet of the animals. A veterinarian should be consulted first before feeding copper.

Copper

Copper may also accumulate in plants in amounts great enough to cause toxic effects if soils are rich in copper or deficient in molybdenum. Clovers are good accumulators of copper and are generally associated with copper poisoning.

Selenium

Selenium is a highly toxic element when taken in quantities larger than what is needed for normal metabolism. In most plants, the level of selenium is related to levels in the soil. The symptoms of selenium poisoning are: dullness, stiffness of joints, lameness, loss of hair from mane or tail and hoof deformities. The acute form of poisoning is often called “blind staggers”.

Ergot

Ergot is a fungus that infests grasses and if eaten in sufficient quantities is poisonous due to the production of a mycotoxin. Ergot’s presence is observed by hard, dark-coloured masses in flowering grass heads. These purplish or dark brown masses are usually two to five times larger than the grass seed and are called ergot bodies.

The active toxin, ergotoxine, stimulates the nerve centres that cause contraction of the small blood vessels supplying the different parts of the body. The result of ergot poisoning depends largely upon the amount of the fungus consumed. When only small quantities have been taken in, recovery without any serious symptoms may take place. Where large quantities have been consumed, dry gangrene in the extremities, possible abortion in pregnant animals and death may result.

General symptoms such as lack of appetite, dullness, abdominal pain, and subnormal temperature are common. Two distinct types of symptoms may develop in severe cases:

Nervous Form

Dullness and depression are evident. There may be muscular trembling, convulsions, contractions of legs, and delirium. The animal suffers from gastrointestinal catarrh, refuses food, and gradually develops a wasting condition. A very rapid type in which the animal may die in spasms or convulsions is sometimes seen.

Gangrenous or General Form

The stoppage of blood due to the contraction of the small blood vessels causes necrosis (death) of the extremities, particularly the feet, the tail, or tips of the ears. The affected part is cool, and dries up; a small furrow or line of separation appears and completely surrounds the limb, dividing the living tissue from the dead. There is little or no loss of blood, and seldom any pus present. Death may also occur due to the invasion of bacterial organisms, "secondary invaders", as well as from gangrene. Cases that do recover may be crippled for life.

The following are some of the crop, pasture and wild grasses on which ergot has been known to develop: oats, barley, wheat, rye, red top, bent grasses, meadow foxtail, brome grasses, orchard grass, reed canary, timothy fescues, blue grasses, quack grass, poverty oat grass, and foxtails.

Mycotoxins

Other mycotoxins are produced by some fungi that infect corn and cereals. The mycotoxins are produced only if the right environmental conditions are met and these conditions vary depending on the fungus.

It is possible for mycotoxin production to take place while the crop is still standing in the field or after it is harvested and in storage.

In Ontario, the two most common forms of mycotoxins are vomitoxin and zearalenone. Vomitoxin causes the animal which eats the contaminated feed to vomit. Usually, however, animals refuse to eat the feed.

Zearalenone is a female estrogen. Symptoms in swine, the class of livestock that is usually affected, are as follows: females show signs of irregular heat, immature gilts develop a marked swelling and inflammation of the external genital organs, reduced litter sizes, and males may lose libido.

Coumarin

Coumarin, a chemical found in sweet clover, is responsible for the reduced palatability of this legume and is associated with a reduced blood clotting ability in the animals who eat sweetclover. Coumarin itself, however, does not cause this latter problem. Dicoumarol, a chemical derived from coumarin, during heating or spoilage of sweet clover hay or silage is the chemical that is responsible. If the clotting ability of the blood is lowered, it is possible that animals may bleed to death from slight wounds, dehorning, castrating or from internal hemorrhages.

Chapter 3

Other Types of Poisoning or Injury to Animals

Photosensitisation

Certain plants contain toxic agents which, when eaten, render the animal sensitive to strong sunlight. The damage that results can range from sunburning and swelling of the sensitive areas to the formation of ulcers and gangrene. Animals may also become blind.

Photosensitisation cases are divided into two groups, primary and hepatogenic. Primary phototoxic plants have toxins that directly photosensitise the skin either through contact or by ingestation. When eaten, the toxins are absorbed and circulated in the blood to the skin where they are activated by the rays of the sun. The unpigmented (white) skin is affected.

The second group, the hepatogenic phototoxic plants, do not directly cause photosensitisation. These plants have toxins that damage the liver. The liver damage prevents a breakdown product of chlorophyll (phylloerythrin) from being removed in the bile fluid. The phylloerythrin is circulated to the capillaries of the skin where it is activated by the sun and produces symptoms similar to those with primary photosensitisation. It is important with hepatogenic cases to treat the damaged liver.

Saint John's-wort, spring parsley and buckwheat cause primary photosensitisation. Blue-green algae causes hepatogenic cases.

Plants Affecting Milk and its Production

Certain plants are known to decrease milk production. They may also make the milk or milk products unpalatable and unsuitable for human consumption. The following lists some of these plants:

- curled dock
- broad-leaved dock

- wild onion
- wild garlic
- buttercup
- marsh marigold
- lupines
- Saint John's-wort
- wild carrot
- burdock
- false flax
- flixweed
- wild mustard
- hedge mustard
- turnips
- rape
- spurges
- buckthorn
- yarrow
- garlic mustard
- stinking mayweed
- ox-eye daisy
- ragweed
- tansy
- absinth
- wormwood
- white snakeroot
- chicory
- stinkweed
- jimson weed.

Algae in Water

Water may contain blue-green algae which can poison livestock. This type of algae is usually found in stagnant or slow-moving water during July and August. Long periods of warm weather and a high content of organic matter in the water favour its growth.

As a general rule, symptoms develop very rapidly and resemble an allergic reaction. Animals may be found dead at the water's edge or after having walked a few metres. Convulsions may occur, but more frequently the animal sinks to the ground, and dies without struggling. Smaller amounts of poison cause weakness and staggering, followed by recovery.

In some instances, apparent recovery from an attack is followed in a few days or weeks by evidence of photosensitisation. There may be innammation of the muzzle, the skin of the ear, the udder, or other parts of the body. Jaundice is often seen, and constipation is a common symptom. Such cases usually recover under good care.

Plants Causing Mechanical Injury

Some plants cause physical or mechanical injury to animals, and this injury may be external or internal. When this occurs, there is also the danger of infection of these injuries which may prove to be even more serious. This is sometimes the case with Canada thistle.

The barbs or awns of foxtail barley, downy brome, and wild rye are often troublesome in the mouths and throats of animals that have fed on these plants. The small, backward-pointing spines cause the awns to stick in the mouth or throat, and they are difficult to dislodge.

The spines of the fruit of the sandbur are quite stiff, and an animal grazing may injure its muzzle while cropping, or if burs get into its mouth they may cause a painful injury.

The burs of cocklebur and burdock, are also a source of annoyance. When the burs are eaten, they form an indigestible ball in the stomach. The spines injure the wall of the digestive tract and may thus open the way for secondary infection.

The sap from some plants, such as the spurges and buttercups, is a source of irritation to the skin of animals. After contact with the plant juices, the skin becomes inflamed and painful blisters may form. This type of damage to the mouth reduces the animal's desire or ability to eat.

Reportable Animal Diseases

The Ministry of Agriculture and Food continually works closely with the Canadian Food Inspection Agency (CFIA) to maintain surveillance and controls and to disseminate information on foreign and reportable animal diseases. This coordinated, overall risk management approach is essential for Canada to rapidly detect reportable livestock diseases and effectively mitigate any negative impacts should they occur.

While the CFIA is the lead agency for all reportable livestock diseases, the provincial government also has a role to play to ensure continued public health, a safe food supply and protection of our agricultural industries. OMAF provides assistance to the CFIA and public health officials in ongoing investigations, as well as offering ongoing stakeholder support through the Ontario Animal Health Surveillance Network, and dairy and meat inspection services.

One of Ontario's biggest monitoring and prevention assets is our strong network of veterinarians-working in private practice, in government and at provincial and federal abattoirs. Veterinarians are highly trained to recognise symptoms of reportable and other animal diseases and know what to do should any suspicious cases arise.

By law, all reportable diseases, including any suspect case, must be immediately reported to a federal veterinarian. Specific control and eradication measures for these diseases are already established and ready to be implemented if needed.

Bioterrorism Involving Livestock

In light of the recent events in North America, governments and the public have a heightened awareness and concern about the possibility of bioterrorism involving agriculture, including livestock. This alert is not meant to cause panic or overstate the obvious. However, veterinarians and livestock owners may be the first to diagnose the early cases of a bioterrorist act in agriculture, as livestock can be sentinels of such an exposure. At the very least this note provides further points of contact for more information.

The Centres for Disease Control and Prevention in the United States has produced a list of the most likely biological agents to be used in an act of bioterrorism. Many of these are pathogens shared by humans and animals, and some have agricultural significance. Other agents of concern include Foreign Animal Diseases and other reportable diseases (such as Foot and Mouth Disease, Avian Influenza). Although many of the pathogens listed as possible bioterrorism agents would cause localised or sporadic disease, some may have serious public health or trade implications. Veterinarians should remain current and vigilant for clinical signs consistent with any reportable or foreign animal disease, as well as unusual patterns or clusters of disease from the agents listed below. The Animal Health Laboratory

(University of Guelph) and other diagnostic laboratories across Canada have been notified to be on alert for the detection of such agents. Diseases or clusters that might point to an exposure consistent with an act of bioterrorism could include: unusual demographic patterns, multiple species involvement, concurrent animal/public health problems, and unusual clusters of strains or serotypes.

Centres for Disease Control and Prevention-Critical Biological Agents

Category A

The U.S. public health system and primary health-care providers must be prepared to address varied biological agents, including pathogens that are rarely seen in the United States. High-priority agents include organisms that pose a risk to national security because they:

- can be easily disseminated or transmitted person-to-person;
- cause high mortality, with potential for major public health impact;
- might cause public panic and social disruption; and
- require special action for public health preparedness.

Category A agents include:

- variola major (smallpox);
- Bacillus anthracis (anthrax);
- Yersinia pestis (plague);
- Clostridium botulinum toxin (botulism);
- Francisella tularensis (tularaemia);
- Filoviruses (e.g. Ebola hemorrhagic fever, Marburg hemorrhagic fever);
- Arenaviruses (c.g. Lassa (Lassa fever), Junin (Argentine hemorrhagic fever)).

Category B

Second highest priority agents include those that:

- are moderately easy to disseminate;
- cause moderate morbidity and low mortality; and
- require specific enhancements of CDC's diagnostic capacity and enhanced disease surveillance.

Category B agents include:

- Coxiella burnetti (Q fever);
- Brucella species (brucellosis);
- Burkholderia mallei (glanders);
- Alphaviruses (e.g. Venezuelan encephalomyelitis, eastren and westren equine encephalomyelitis);
- Venezuelan encephalomyelitis;
- ricin toxin from Ricinus communis (castor beans);
- epsilon toxin of Clostridium perfringens;
- Staphylococcus enterotoxin B;
- Chlamydia psittaci (Psittacosis)

A subset of List B agents includes pathogens that are food or waterborne. These pathogens include but are not limited to:

- Salmonella species;
- Shigella dysenteriae;
- Escherichia coli O157:H7;
- Vibrio cholerae; and
- Cryptosporidium parvum.

Category C

Third highest priority agents include emerging pathogens that could be engineered for mass dissemination in the future because of:

- availability;
- ease of production and dissemination; and
- potential for high morbidity and mortality and major health impact.

Category C agents include:

- Nipah virus;
- hantaviruses;
- tickborne hemorrhagic fever viruses;
- tickborne encephalitis viruses;
- yellow fever; and
- multidrug-resistant tuberculosis.

Rabies

Cause and Transmission

- Rabies is caused by a virus (Lyssavirus).
- It can infect all warm-blooded animals, including humans.
- The animals that most often transmit infection in Canada are foxes, raccoons, skunks and bats.
- Usually spread by saliva that contains the virus, often by the bite of an infected animal.
- More rarely, virus from saliva can be introduced into open cuts or wounds. Saliva can also infect by contact with a mucous membrane (mouth, nasal cavity, eyes).
- Raccoon rabies poses the same risks as rabies in other animals-the only difference is that it is spread primarily by raccoons.

Occurance

- Rabies is a reportable disease-if an animal is suspected of being rabid or an animal(s) has been exposed to rabies, it is the law to report it.
- Call your nearest office of the Canadian Food Inspection Agency (CFIA), which is listed in the blue pages of the phone book-an inspector from the agency will investigate all calls.
- The wildlife baiting (vaccination) program of the Ontario Ministry of Natural Resources has dramatically decreased the level of rabies in the province-but the risk is not zero.
- Pockets of rabies can occur depending on the wildlife ecology of the area.

Clinical Signs

- Incubation period varies from 2 weeks to several months.
- Clinical signs are highly variable.

Cattle

- yawning, bellowing, incoordination, decreased feeling in hindlimbs, loss of tail movement, drooling saliva, "cud-dropping", inability to stand, hypersensitivity, aggression, paralysis

Sheep

- sexual excitement, wool pulling, aggression, incoordination, paralysis

Horses

- abnormal postures, lameness, weakness, depression, muscle incoordination, inability to swallow, inability to stand, biting, aggression, hypersensitivity, loss of anal tone

Pigs

- excitement, aggression, twitching of nose, convulsions, paralysis

Dogs and Cats

- changes in behaviour, depression, hypersensitivity, aggression, muscle incoordination, changes in vocalisation, excessive salivation, paralysis

Wildlife

- show no fear of man, aggression, incoordination, active during the day instead of at night
- Remember that the most typical thing about rabies is that it can be atypical.

Treatment

- None-rabies is fatal once clinical signs appear.
- If an animal is bitten or comes in contact with a suspected rabies case, contact a veterinarian or the Canadian Food Inspection Agency immediately.
- If a person is bitten by an animal, wash the wound or exposed surface with soap and water, remove clothing that may be contaminated, contact your doctor immediately or go to the nearest hospital emergency room.
- Post-exposure treatment for people is effective and low risk, but expensive.

Prevention

- Vaccinate pets and livestock-this keeps your pets and livestock from getting rabies, but also provides a barrier of protection to humans.
- Vaccination for rabies is good insurance and an inexpensive way of protecting your livestock and pets, as well as your family and friends.
- Ask your veterinarian about the type and frequency of rabies vaccination.

- Enjoy wild animals (raccoons, skunks, foxes) from afar-do not handle, feed, or unintentionally attract wild animals (secure garbage cans).
- Do not approach animals showing abnormal behaviour.
- Never adopt wild animals or bring them into your home-do not try to nurse sick animals to health.
- Teach children never to approach and handle unfamiliar animals, wild or domestic, even if they appear friendly.

Pig Farms for Diseases of Public Health Significance

The food industry is vulnerable to concerns regarding human health risks, whether the issues are real or a result of media hype. Consumers are demanding monitoring programs that evaluate food safety risks from the farm through to the retail outlet. A number of diseases that can move from pig to people are best minimised by programs directed at the farm level. Some of Canada's major competitors have undertaken on-farm monitoring programs as a means to improve the quality and safety of their product and to ensure the expansion of their world market share. In order for Ontario to institute a program of monitoring and to develop strategies to reduce human pathogens at the farm level, it is first necessary to investigate what the true prevalence of disease is and what the limitations of the current testing procedure are.

Approximately 100 producers from farms all over southern Ontario have participated in this large scale surveillance project. A long list of potential disease agents have been tested for including *Salmonella*, *Yersinia*, *Toxoplasma*, *Swine Influenza virus*, *E. coli* 0157:H7 and intestinal parasites like *Balantidium coli*, *Giardia* and *Cryptosporidia*. In addition, drug use and the presence of drug resistance was measured.

Not surprising, all of the above organisms were either isolated or antibodies to them (indicating exposure) were found in at least a few herds. For some diseases like *Toxoplasmosis*, the presence of antibodies indicating a positive animal was lower than has been found in previous studies indicating that modern husbandry practices are reducing the risk of disease. The presence of cats on a farm is a major risk factor for pigs to become infected with *Toxoplasma*, and new operations seldom rely on cats for rodent control whereas a high proportion of older facilities have cats present.

Larger and new facilities often use all-in/all-out management with cleaning and disinfection between groups of pigs. This procedure appears to reduce the risk of bacterial pathogens such as *Yersinia enterocolitica. Yersiniosis* is a common cause of food-poisoning in humans and pigs are likely the major source of infection so that it is a disease that the pork industry needs to be aware of and monitor closely.

Most experts consider *Salmonellosis* is as the most important issue facing the pig industry as far as food safety. The challenge in monitoring *Salmonella* is deciding what test to use and how to interpret the results. Culturing techniques that work satisfactorily in detecting sick animals are not very sensitive in identifying subclinical carrier animals.

There are more elaborate culturing techniques which use several enrichment steps that be used to find more *Salmonella* but at a great cost and are time consuming. Europeans use serological tests to measure antibodies as a means of screening herds for the presence of *Salmonella*.

This can be much quicker and cheaper than culturing. The UofG study suggests that unless the serological tests are modified to include more strains of *Salmonella*, there will be herds where *Salmonella* can be grown from pigs but the herd will test negative on serology. If Ontario decides to institute a program similar to Denmark where pork producers whose pigs test positive for *Salmonella* are penalised, then these issues regarding testing will need to be addressed.

A major accomplishment of this surveillance study is that we now have a good idea as to the prevalence of this group of diseases on Ontario farms and an idea of how widespread they are when they are present on a farm.

Q Fever

Q fever is a zoonotic disease, usually associated with ruminants, caused by the rickettsia Coxiella burnetii. It has been reported throughout most of the world, including Canada. In Ontario, Q fever has occasionally been diagnosed as a cause of abortion in sheep and goats. Reported human cases have been associated with exposure to abortions in sheep and goats, and drinking unpasteurised goat's milk.

Most human infections with C. burnetii are asymptomatic or result in only a mild transient flu-like illness. Infection in animals is common, and also largely asymptomatic. In North America, clinical disease is usually limited to abortion in sheep and goats, but cattle are thought to be a significant source of human exposure.

Source of Infection and Mode of Transmission

The reservoirs of infection include wild and domestic mammals, birds and arthropods such as ticks. Serologic studies suggest that infection may be widespread in the animal population, but the real prevalence is unknown. The prevalence will also vary considerably across species, geographic location and time. Studies in Ontario have found evidence of C. burnetii infection in 33-82% of cattle herds and 0-35% of sheep flocks. Cattle, sheep and goats are considered the main source of infection to humans.

The rickettsial agent becomes localised in the mammary glands and placenta of infected ruminants, and is excreted in large numbers in milk, placental tissue, fetal fluids, urine and feces. Consequently, parturition can result in significant environmental contamination and is likely the time of greatest risk for transmission of the disease within herds and flocks, and to humans. Dogs and cats may also be infected and shed the rickettsia. Exposure to placenta and contaminated materials from cats has been a common source of human Q fever infection in Nova Scotia.

C. burnetii is very resistant to environmental and chemical factors, and may persist in the environment for several weeks. The main route of Q fever infection in humans is by aerosol transmission, either directly from the placenta and fetal fluids of infected animals or from contaminated wool, hides or bedding. The organism can be transported long distances on dust particles, and some windborne outbreaks have been documented. Despite the presence of the agent in raw milk, clinical infection through the digestive tract in North America is thought to be rare. Ticks may play a role in the natural cycle of infection in wildlife populations, but human disease associated with tick bites has only occasionally been documented.

Chapter 4

Infection in Animals and Humans

Naturally infected animals do not show any clinical signs of disease, including fever, at the time of infection. The udder and uterus are the main sites of infection, with large numbers of the organism being shed in the milk and birth materials. The infection can become chronic, reoccurring at subsequent parturition.

Human Q fever is primarily an occupational disease of farmers, abattoir workers, veterinarians, and laboratory workers. In the majority of cases the disease is a non-specific flu-like illness with a 1-3 week incubation period, often remaining undiagnosed. In a minority of cases there will be a clinical atypical pneumonia or hepatitis. Should the course of disease become chronic, endocarditis and chronic hepatitis can develop. Chronic Q fever is often fatal, and may be more likely to develop in immunocompromised individuals and pregnant women.

Treatment

In animals, once C. burnetii has been identified as the cause of an abortion, the rest of the flock or herd can be protected to some degree by the use of long acting injectable tetracyclines. Acute human clinical cases generally respond to appropriate antibiotic therapy. Treatment of the chronic condition has been less successful, with relapses common.

Precautions

1. In assisting any aborting or parturient animal, it is advisable to wear protective clothing, disposable gloves and a mask covering the mouth and nose. Pregnant women or the immunocompromised should not assist in the birthing of animals.
2. Aborting animals should be isolated for 3 weeks. As an extra precaution the hindquarters can be washed to remove any residual organisms. All placental tissue and contaminated

material such as bedding should be removed and destroyed, preferably by burning or composting, and the pen thoroughly cleaned and disinfected before being used again. The most effective disinfectant against C. burnetti is a 1:100 lysol solution. Even dogs and cats should be allowed to deliver in isolation on disposable bedding.

3. Unpasteurised milk must not be consumed. The recommended time for home pasteurisation is 30 minutes at 63° C or 15 seconds at 72° C (5).

Bovine Tuberculosis (Mycobacterium Bovis)

Bovine Tuberculosis is a contagious, debilitating disease of both humans and animals. It is caused by the bacterium Mycobacterium bovis (M. bovis), part of the Mycobacterium complex which also includes M. tuberculosis and M. avium. The primary site of infection is the lymph nodes, but spread to other organs such as the lungs will occur as the disease progresses. Clinical signs of the disease include weakness, loss of appetite, weight loss and fever. Bovine TB is a chronic disease, and infected animals may take several years to develop clinical signs or may show no evidence of infection until they are sent to slaughter.

Cattle are the usual host for M. bovis, but bovine TB can be transmitted to humans as well as other animals such as swine, bison and cervids (deer and elk). The bacteria do not survive exposure to heat, sunlight or dry conditions, and do not replicate outside the host. People at greatest risk are those in direct and prolonged contact with infected animals, such as farmers, farm workers and veterinarians. The most common means of contracting the disease is through inhalation of aerosols containing TB bacteria exhaled or coughed out by an infected animal. The risk of exposure is greatest in enclosed areas such as barns. Other methods of exposure include the drinking of unpasteurised milk from an infected cow and the sharing of common water or feed sources.

Because the disease in cattle may not be clinically evident, even in advanced stages, diagnosis is often made upon post mortem examination at slaughter. Nodular lesions may be found in any organ or body cavity, but are usually seen in the lungs and associated lymph nodes of the head, respiratory and gastrointestinal tracts.

In Canada, Bovine Tuberculosis is a reportable disease under the Health of Animals Act. When a veterinarian reports a suspected case, the Canadian Food Inspection Agency follows a strict testing and eradication program. Preliminary diagnosis of TB infection is through the tuberculin skin test. This confirms exposure to a type of Mycobacterium but further diagnostic methods are necessary to confirm the presence of bovine TB. In humans, this includes chest x-rays and sputum cultures.

For cattle, a diagnosis is normally made through post mortem examination and tissue culture, although bacterial culture to confirm the presence of M. bovis can take up to 12 weeks. Once bovine TB is confirmed, all infected and exposed animals are destroyed with federal compensation. After the premises have been depopulated, the owner is responsible for cleaning and disinfecting the facility under CFIA guidance.

Livestock and Poultry Diseases

Ontario is moving to protect animal and human health, and the economic viability of the livestock and poultry sector, by reducing the impact of animal diseases.

The proposed Animal Health Act, 2009 *was introduced in the Ontario legislature today. The legislation, if passed, would:*

- provide measures to assist in the prevention, detection, response to and control of animal diseases and other hazards to protect the livestock and poultry sector
- require the reporting of specific animal diseases to the Chief Veterinarian for Ontario
- enable the use of quarantine orders, surveillance zones and animal health control area orders to help control the spread of any detected disease or hazard
- support a future traceability framework for the quick identification and control of disease and food safety hazards.

Quotes

This proposed legislation would protect both animal and human health and would enable us to respond to disease situations promptly. Protecting livestock and poultry is important for the economic well-being of the industry and for all of Ontario." — Leona Dombrowsky, Minister of Agriculture, Food and Rural Affairs

"The proposed legislation allows us to better prepare for and respond to animal health issues. This would be yet another step in strengthening Ontario's animal health system, which benefits us all." — Dr. Deb Stark, Chief Veterinarian for Ontario

"The Ontario Livestock and Poultry Council members are very pleased that the Ontario government is moving forward with animal health legislation. We feel the proposed Act will provide the provincial government and the livestock and poultry industry with the required tools to reduce the likelihood of a major disease occurrence and assist with controlling its spread if one should occur." — Gord Coukell, Chair, Ontario Livestock and Poultry Council

"OVMA welcomes and supports the Ontario government in proposing a modern framework for the protection and promotion of animal health in Ontario. As veterinary practitioners, we are front-line health care professionals committed to protecting Ontario's agri-food industry, animal and human health from the negative impacts associated with animal-borne diseases through effective disease surveillance and detection, and improved traceability and biosecurity measures."

The Diseases and Parasites of Farmed Cervids

Bacterial Diseases

Brucellosis or *B. abortus* causes abortions, arthritis and debilitating disease in Bovidae and Cervidae, and undulant fever in people (Smits, 1991; Radostits et al., 1994). Brucellosis is a named disease under the Animal Health Act, therefore control and eradication falls under the jurisdiction of the Canadian Food Inspection Agency (CFIA). Brucellosis was declared eradicated from the Canadian domestic cattle herd in 1985, and the only known reservoir of Brucellosis in Canada, is bison in Wood Buffalo National Park (Tessaro et al., 1993).

Brucellosis is not endemic in wild deer in Canada, nor has it been recognised in farmed deer, tested under CFIA's Captive Ungulate Program. Brucellosis does occur in wild elk in certain refuges in Wyoming, as a result of a spill over of infection from cattle and bison in the Yellow stone National Park region. Its transmission is promoted by congregation associated with winter feeding of elk. Brucellosis is transmitted mainly by ingestion of organisms shed in body secretions and in the fetal fluids of abortuses.

Status in Canada/Ontario

Brucellosis is endemic in bison in Wood Buffalo National Park, but has been eradicated in cattle and is not present in any species in Ontario.

Species: Cattle, bison, elk can become persistently infected carriers, and under appropriate circumstances of population size, density and management, can develop endemic disease. Other deer are susceptible to infection, but apparently rarely develop endemic infections in populations, or clinical disease. The exception is moose, which get severe disease and may die, but as a result, are unlikely to be able to sustain an endemic disease state in a population (Forbes et al., 1996).

Probability of Entry/Transmission/Endemicity

Low, given efficacy of import testing, rejection at import of animals from infected herds, and CFIA's ongoing testing as part of the Captive Ungulate Program. Brucellosis is unlikely to establish in wild deer in Ontario, based on experience in USA and Ontario, when Brucellosis was common in cattle, and deer were presumably exposed from that source.

Control/Mitigation

CFIA control and test imported animals and domestic farmed deer under the Captive Ungulate Program. As noted earlier Brucellosis is a named disease and therefore control and eradication falls under the jurisdiction of the Canadian Food Inspection Agency, formerly Agriculture Canada. Eradication has been successful in cattle, and would seem feasible in farmed deer, if the disease were identified. The control of Brucellosis would be difficult in an infected population of susceptible wildlife, without the feasibility of eradication.

Key components to the control of Brucellosis include conformity CFIA regulations, proper animal identification and inventory records, and the containment of farmed deer.

Johne's Disease (ParaTuberculosis)

Johne's disease is caused by Mycobacterium avium paraTuberculosis. All species of ruminants, including deer (Smits, 1991; Haigh and Hudson, 1993), as well as camelids (Stehman, 1996), rabbits (Greig et al., 1997) and some other species are assumed to be susceptible. The disease is common in domestic cattle, sheep, goats and farmed deer (eg. Power et al., 1993; Fawcett et al., 1995) over most of the world, including Ontario (McNab et al., 1991), where it has been diagnosed in farmed fallow and sika deer (Barker, Hazlett and Ernst, 1997).

The organism is transmitted via close contact/ingestion, or transplacentally, from dam to fetus (Sweeney, 1996). The incubation period is long, from perhaps 6-10 months in some species of deer, to about 2 years or more in cattle and sheep. It causes granulomatous enteritis and lymphadenitis, resulting in weight loss progressing to emaciation, and in many species, diarrhea (Clarke, 1997). Reduced productivity and premature loss of the animal due to death contribute to the cost of this disease.

Johne's disease has apparently been transmitted from domestic animals to wildlife in several areas of North America: bighorn sheep and Rocky Mountain goats in the Rocky Mountain states (Williams et al., 1983); Tule elk in California (Jessup et al., 1981; Cook et al., 1997); white-tailed deer in the northeastern US (Libke and Walton, 1975; Chiodini and VanKruiningen, 1983), and free-living fallow and axis deer (Reimann et al., 1979).

Status in Canada/Ontario

Johne's Disease is endemic in conventional domestic ruminants and in farmed deer

Species: All species of farmed and wild ruminants, including all species of deer

Probability of Entry/Transmission/Endemicity

Moderate: The probability of spreading and becoming endemic in wild deer populations is difficult to determine. It is fairly common in domestic animals, but has yet to be recognised in wild deer in Ontario. High deer densities or congregations might promote development of endemic Johne's disease. Farmed deer probably add little incremental risk to that already posed by infected conventional domestic ruminants in Ontario.

Degree of Harm: Moderate: The disease is insidious, and if it established, might cause incremental mortality in wild populations, that could be difficult to detect or recognise. Population effects on wildlife unstudied.

Overall Risk: Moderate, but farmed deer probably add little incremental risk to that already posed by infected conventional domestic ruminants in Ontario.

Control/Mitigation

Tests for the infection in the living animal are unreliable and insensitive (Stehmann, 1996), and so disease control by test and slaughter is not feasible. Surveillance via autopsies on animals sick or dying on farm will detect the disease. There is a slight possibility of confusion of paraTuberculosis with Tuberculosis at autopsy; both are caused by Mycobacterium (but different species), and they should be differentiated by culture or molecular probes if there is any doubt about the diagnosis. Deer farmers should attempt to purchase stock from farms with a veterinary certificate, indicting no history of Johne's Disease, to prevent its spread in the industry.

Management issues relating to control/mitigation of Johne's Disease include the confinement of farmed deer, a herd health program and autopsies of animals dying on farm.

Tuberculosis (Mycobacterium bovis)

Deer are susceptible to bovine Tuberculosis, caused by the bacterium Mycobacterium bovis, which produces a debilitating disease in a proportion of infected animals (Griffin and Buchan, 1994), and can be transmitted to people (Fanning and Edwards, 1991; Grange and Yates, 1994; Liss et al., 1994). Tuberculosis is a named disease under the Animal Health Act and therefore falls under the jurisdiction of CFIA. With the approaching eradication of this disease from the Canadian cattle herd (Essey and Koller, 1994), Tuberculosis in farmed deer assumes significance for four major reasons: health problems in deer; possibility of transmission back into the cattle population; possibility of transmission to wildlife; and the possibility of transmission to people. In most countries, deer have been a secondary agricultural species, and subsequently resources applied to Tuberculosis control programs centred first on the primary species of concern, cattle. This was also the case in Canada. The upsurge of interest in deer farming in the late 1980's, and associated international trade in deer, exposed weaknesses in standard testing protocols, which had worked well in detecting Tuberculosis-infected cattle, but had relatively low sensitivity in deer (Griffin and Buchan, 1994). As a result, bovine Tuberculosis became an obvious problem in a variety of countries in North America and western Europe, as international and internal trade in deer mushroomed.

Depopulation of deer herds with Tuberculosis had been ongoing sporadically, but in 1988, Agriculture Canada (now CFIA) established the Captive Ungulate Program, aimed at systematically testing all herds of non-domestic ungulates in the country for Tuberculosis and Brucellosis, with the goal of eradicating these diseases in that segment of the animal population. Testing under this program began in Ontario in 1990.

Tuberculosis in deer may be detected three ways: by skin testing as part of the Captive Ungulate Program; by detection of lesions in tissue during meat inspection at an abattoir (all legal abattoirs in

Ontario must be inspected under either provincial OMAF regulations, or under federal CFIA regulations); or if a veterinarian suspects a diagnosis of Tuberculosis (eg. at autopsy, which has occurred several times in Ontario).

Tuberculosis (TB) has been detected on a number of bison, deer and elk farms, and in zoos and menageries in Canada. Most cases seem ultimately to be traceable to the importation of elk from the USA, prior to revision of the cervid TB test protocol, with one possibly attributable to the import of deer from New Zealand. Imports of deer from these countries have not been permitted since 1990/91. In Ontario, 10 premises with Tuberculous deer were detected and depopulated by Agriculture Canada between January 1990 and November 1994. No premises with confirmed Tuberculosis in deer have been detected in Ontario since that time. However, an estimate of over 5,100 deer on about 150 premises (30% and 45% of provincial totals of deer and farms, respectively) remain untested in Ontario as of March 1998. These 150 premises include deer farms as well as non-farm operations such as zoos, menageries, parks and petting zoos.

"Restricted" status herds remain untested for a variety of reasons, mainly related to an absence of satisfactory handling facilities. There is consequently difficulty in reading tests, and physical danger to the CFIA veterinarian, the animals and their handlers, posed by testing under inadequate circumstances (eg. by drug immobilisation of unrestrained animals using syringe dart guns etc.). Drug immobilisation of deer by syringe dart is expensive. TB testing requires reading skin tests within a specific time frame, good lighting, a clean skin test site and the ability to identify the animal accurately and keep records. This is difficult in an unsheltered paddock, especially if animals are difficult to apprehend reliably and restrain adequately.

Tuberculosis has rarely been reported from free-ranging cervids anywhere in the world. Tuberculosis is known to be established in wildlife in Canada, only in bison in Wood Buffalo National Park (Essey and Koller, 1994). Hadwen (1942) reported Tuberculosis in elk, mule deer and moose in Alberta. A single Tuberculous elk was encountered in the vicinity of a farm with TB-infected cattle in Manitoba (Rhyan et al., 1992) and a single case was reported in a white-tailed deer from Ontario (Belli, 1962). Sporadic cases of TB have also been reported in wild cervids in the USA. With the exception of the single Ontario white-tailed deer, all cases listed were in association with Tuberculosis in farmed animals, including farmed elk, or feral swine (Rhyan et al., 1995).

In 1994, a population of white-tailed deer with endemic bovine Tuberculosis was identified in northeastern Michigan (Schmitt et al., 1997). The origin of the infection in this population is unclear, and its duration is unknown, although a Tuberculous deer was reported in the vicinity in 1975 (Schmitt et al, 1997). Michigan at one time had a very high prevalence of Tuberculosis in cattle (Schmitt et al., 1997), and it is probable that the disease spilled over into deer decades ago, and went unrecognised. It seems unlikely that it originated with farmed deer, since only one case of TB has been identified in farmed cervids in Michigan, despite extensive surveillance (Michigan DNR, c. 1997), and the genetic fingerprint of M. bovis isolated from wild white-tailed deer resembles that of cattle isolates, and is dissimilar from the Michigan elk isolate (Whipple et al., 1998).

Tuberculosis is a density-dependent disease in ruminants, since close contact promotes successful transmission, mainly by the respiratory route, or by ingestion (Radostits et al., 1994). Variations in herd behaviour and density have been invoked to explain differences in prevalence of Tuberculosis in wild cervids. Hadwen (1942) considered that elk, as herd animals, were more prone to transmission of TB than mule deer, and Schmitt et al. (1997) suggest that artificial feeding, with attendant close contact among animals, may be the factor which has permitted Tuberculosis to remain endemic in wild deer in the affected area of Michigan.

A computer model suggests that the rate of transmission among deer will have to drop by more than 50% before the prevalence of the disease will begin to decline (Corso et al., 1997). Michigan initially proposed attempting to reduce transmission by voluntary restrictions on supplementary winter feeding and by increasing hunting pressure (Schmitt et al., 1997). However, more recently, they have initiated stringent compulsory restrictions on feeding deer in the affected area (Anony mous, 1998c).

While white-tailed deer densities in Ontario do not approach those in the affected area of Michigan. Supplementary winter feeding on deer yards might set up circumstances favourable for maintenance of Tuberculosis in a local population in this province, were the disease introduced, especially if escaped farmed deer commingled with wild.

Status in Canada/Ontario

Probability of Entry/Transmission/Endemicity

Low probability of entry currently, due to CFIA testing (cattle) or non-issuance of permits for imports (deer). Moderate to high probability of transmission and subsequent endemicity in wildlife, while potentially infected deer remain in the farmed population

Control/Mitigation

Universal and full compliance with the CFIA's control program is the key to controlling, mitigating and eventually eradicating Tuberculosis from the deer farming industry. Important components of the CFIA's Captive Ungulate Program include import testing/ controls, on-farm testing and eradication, and movement controls. Other important elements contributing to the success of the control program include adequate animal identification and deer inventory records, as well as proper on-farm containment of deer.

Yersiniosis

Yersiniosis is caused by enteric bacteria of the genus Yersinia, mainly Y. pseudotuberculosis. Yersiniosis is a disease predominantly of red deer, though it also occurs in other species of deer, and in sheep and cattle (Haigh and Hudson, 1993; Radostits et al., 1994; Sanford, 1995; Diseases Diagnosed at Autopsy in Farmed Deer in Ontario, Barker, Hazlett and Ernst).

The organism is present in soil, water and feces, and strains with particular virulence attributes invade the intestinal mucosa, causing diarrhea, weight loss, and sometimes systemic infection. Losses can be severe in farmed deer, and treatment is difficult. The disease is most common in stressed weaners in their first fall, when adverse weather conditions seem able to precipitate outbreaks (Sanford, 1995). Yersiniosis is a sporadic disease in a variety of wild mammals and birds other than deer, causing mortality in beaver and musk-ox, among other species, but apparently has not been recognised in free-ranging deer in Ontario.

Status in Canada/Ontario

Probability of Entry/Transmission/Endemicity

Low, difficult to determine if effect of deer farming is additive, given that the agent is in the environment in the wild.

Degree of harm: Moderate. The probability of overt disease is slight, but outbreaks may occur.

Control/Mitigation

Ensuring deer remain on-farm (containment) and limiting environmental contamination (manure runoff) are best management practices that will assist in controlling the spread of Yersiniosis.

Viral Diseases

Adenovirus Infections

Adenoviruses are common infectious agents of ungulates, often causing subclinical infection, but occasionally producing respiratory or gastrointestinal disease, or hemorrhagic syndromes, due to replication in vascular endothelium (Mattson, 1992). Antibodies to adenoviruses have been detected in several species of deer (Haigh and Hudson, 1993).

Adenovirus infections have been diagnosed in red deer (Horner and Read, 1982) and fallow deer (Boros et al., 1985), but in neither species can adenoviruses be considered a significant cause of disease. In 1993 an epidemic of adeno virus infection caused high mortality among free-ranging mule deer in northern California (Woods et al., 1996, 1997). The viruses involved are incompletely characterised, and their epidemiology in deer is undefined, though adenoviruses generally are transmitted by close contact or by environmental contamination in other species.

Status in Canada/Ontario

Probability of Entry/Transmission/Endemicity

Moderate/high; infection may be endemic, but is unrecognised in some farmed species. The current infection status of wild cervids in Ontario is unknown.

Moderate: The California outbreak, though regionally significant, appears to have been transient, with no long-term after-effects reported.

Control/Mitigation

Seropositive animals are likely recovered, and not shedding virus; seronegative animals are either uninfected or incubating, so serologic testing to exclude animals carrying the virus is difficult. Control entry of susceptible species; in theory, quarantine and exclude lots of deer which seroconvert in quarantine. There are no controls currently in place.

Adenovirus infections are not considered sufficiently significant in domestic ungulates to warrant specific control measures or vaccination (Mattson, 1992); in fact they are not even considered as a disease problem in the major text on large animal veterinary medicine (Radostits et al., 1994). The containment of farmed deer would reduce, but not eliminate, whatever probability there is, of transmission to wildlife

Bluetongue

An orbivirus infection of ruminants, transmitted by Culicoides midges (certain strains of C. variipennis in North America), endemic in the southern USA, periodically epidemic in the western states (occasionally spilling over into the Okanagan Valley in BC [Sterritt and Dulac, 1992; Dulac et al., 1992]) and mid-eastern states, but not those abutting the border in Ontario (Walton et al., 1992). The virus does not appear to over-winter in arthropods, and the disease dies out as the vector arthropods die in fall/winter (Radostits et al., 1994).

Status in Canada/Ontario

Exotic, with periodic incursions at long intervals into south-central British Columbia (last in 1987-Shapiro et al., 1991); has never been recognised in Ontario.

Species: Cattle are the major reservoir. Goats and elk can be sub-clinical carriers, though wapiti may develop very mild signs. Odocoileus spp., pronghorns and bighorn sheep may develop fatal hemorrhagic disease, but the effect on red deer is unknown (Hoff and Trainer, 1981; Haigh and Hudson, 1993).

Entry/Transmission/Endemicity

Entry could be via infected cattle or elk, not detected by serologic screening, but this is an unlikely event. Entry of this disease by regulated animal imports is not considered significant (Gibbs, 1992). Disease is now recognised as regionalised with respect to risk, based on origin of animal in North America (Walton et al., 1992). This recognises the fact that the disease has never been reported from some areas, and the agent does not over-winter in vectors in the north. Controls are placed by the Canadian Food Inspection Agency on animal movements from infected areas, until risk is deemed negligible, based on vector activity and incubation/transmission period (Sterritt and Dulac, 1992).

It could also enter by wind-borne transportation of vector from south. Local transmission would require presence of suitable vector; the subspecies of C. variipennis in Ontario may be an incompetent vector (Walton et al., 1992). Based on experience in northwestern American states, infected vectors likely would not persist over winter in Ontario, resulting in a transient epidemic impact if the disease did occur. Farmed deer (elk) pose essentially no incremental probability of introduction of Bluetongue to Ontario, beyond the already very low probability posed by importation of cattle and by wind-borne vectors.

Control/Mitigation

CFIA controls the imports into Canada from the USA, based on source, season, and serologic status of herd of origin. There are no other issues directly relevant to BMPs for farmed deer, other than conformity to CFIA regulations and animal identification.

Chronic Wasting Disease (CWD) of Deer and Elk

A prion-associated transmissible spongiform encephalopathy analogous to scrapie in sheep, bovine spongiform encephalopathy (BSE), transmissible mink encephalopathy, and Creutzfeldt-Jakob Disease and Kuru of people. CWD was first described in mule deer in 1980 (Williams and Young, 1980), but had been recognised as a clinical syndrome since 1967 (Williams and Young, 1992). Animals develop behavioural changes, increased drinking/urination, excess salivation and difficulty swallowing, occasionally some ataxia, and in all cases, loss of body condition progressing to emaciation.

The pattern is sporadic, and the minimum incubation period seems to be about 18 months in mule deer and elk. Transmission is horizontal, by contact, and possibly vertical/maternal, from dam to offspring, even with minimum contact after birth. The disease has been recognised in wild elk, mule deer and white-tailed deer in Colorado and Wyoming (Spraker et al., 1997), and in captive elk, mule deer and mule x white-tailed deer hybrids in research facilities and zoos in Colorado, Wyoming and Ontario which had exchanged animals during the 1960's and 1970's (Williams and Young, 1992).

The disease in Ontario involved a small herd of black-tailed/mule deer at the Toronto Zoo, established in the mid-1970's. This herd had connections to a zoo in Colorado in which a syndrome compatible with CWD occurred, and which had exchanged animals with other affected facilities. Animals gradually succumbed to a syndrome compatible with CWD during the late 1970's; the herd died out and was not replaced. A spongiform encephalopathy was diagnosed histologically in one case that died in 1978 (Barker, unpublished), but the syndrome of emaciation was not associated with the spongiform encephalopathy until CWD was described by Williams and Young (1980). Spongiform encephalopathy has not been recognised in any species at the Toronto Zoo since (Barker, unpublished).

The origin of CWD is unknown. There is no clear epidemiologic association with spongiform encephalopathies of domestic animals. Since the affected captive herds were established with wild animals prior to recognition of the disease in free-ranging animals, it is possible that CWD was introduced from the wild population, where it was unknown at the time. This may have occurred following depopulation and re-population of one of these facilities with wild animals in an attempt to eradicate the disease (Williams and Young, 1992). However, surplus animals from affected captive herds had been released to the wild, prior to definition of the disease (Williams and Young, 1992), possibly introducing CWD to the wild population.

CWD was diagnosed in January 1996 in Saskatchewan in a farmed elk which had been imported from South Dakota, USA in 1989. The Saskatchewan herd was depopulated and the first generation progeny of the affected elk which had moved to other farms were also destroyed under Agriculture and Agri-Food Canada supervision (Agriculture and Agri-Food Canada, 1997). As a result of compulsory reporting of illness in farmed deer, required by state regulations, CWD has subsequently been recognised on 2 elk farms in South Dakota, where control measures are underway (Anonymous, 1998a, b).

Status in Canada/Ontario

CWD has not been reported in wild cervids in Canada. CWD is currently not recognised, but has occurred in captive animals in Saskatchewan and Ontario. CFIA, in consultation with Canadian Venison Council, has formulated a policy of surveillance and eradication, though CWD is not a "named disease" under the Health of Animals Act.

Species: Mule deer, white-tailed deer, mule deer x white-tailed deer hybrid, elk are susceptible. The susceptibility of other Cervidae is unknown.

Probability of Entry/Transmission/Endemicity

High in the absence of effective antemortem tests, unless moderated by effective federal import controls (currently in place) and surveillance/eradication program. At the time of the triennial Tuberculosis test, CFIA veterinarians observe captive cervids for signs of disease compatible with CWD (Agriculture and Agri-Food Canada, 1997). Some further infected animals may have entered Canada before the current ban on importation of farmed cervids from USA, and gone undetected. They, the progeny or contacts may be present on farms in Canada.

Control/Mitigation

CFIA control/ban on imports from regions of endemic or unknown status with respect to presence of CWD (currently in place via effective ban on farmed deer imports from USA until import protocols developed [Agriculture and Agri-Food Canada, 1997]). Control/mitigation factors include the on-farm containment of deer, CFIA traceback (identification) and eradication under Captive Ungulate Program and the implementation of an effective internal surveillance for CWD in farmed animals, including the necropsy of deaths.

Epizootic Hemorrhagic Disease (EHD)

This disease is caused by an orbivirus closely related to Bluetongue virus. The two viruses often cocirculate (Shapiro et al., 1991), and the diseases are indistinguishable without virus isolation. It is transmitted by Culicoides midges (certain strains of C. variipennis in northern latitudes), endemic in the southern USA, periodically epidemic in the western and mid-eastern states. Three incursions into Canada are known, in the Cypress Hills area of southern Alberta in 1962; in the Okanagan Valley of BC in 1987 (Sellers and Maarouf, 1991; Shapiro et al, 1991); and on the basis of antibody in cattle, but no disease, in southern Saskatchewan in 1988 (Dulac et al., 1992). The virus does not appear to over-winter in arthropods, and the disease dies out as the vector arthropods die in fall/winter.

Status in Canada/Ontario

The disease is exotic to Canada, with rare incursions into western Canada at long intervals. EHD has never been recognised in Ontario.

Species: A variety of domestic and wild ruminants likely form the reservoir in the southern United States. The disease is rarely recognised in domestic animals. Among wildlife, white-tailed deer are especially susceptible to EHD, while other species, including elk, may develop mild or subclinical disease.

Probability of Entry/Transmission/Endemicity

Low to negligible. EHD is not listed for import control by CFIA under Health of Animals Act, since there is little risk to domestic ruminants, and specific testing is not carried out, though the virus cross-reacts with bluetongue. Entry to Canada is most probable via wind-blown infected vectors from the south (Sellers and Maarouf, 1991).

The epidemiology and risk with respect to vectors in Ontario, is like Bluetongue. Farmed deer pose little incremental probability of introduction of EHD to Ontario, beyond the already very low probability posed by importation of domestic ruminants and by wind-borne vectors.

Control/Mitigation

There is no practical means of control.

"Herpesviruses"

Herpesvirus infections are ubiquitous among ruminants. In cervids, infections occur with "herpesviruses apparently native to deer, and with the sheep or wildebeeste origin (herpesviruses, which cause malignant catarrhal fever.

Alpha herpesviruses of ruminants typically cause mucosal infections and may produce latency in neurons (Engels and Ackermann, 1996). Two "herpesviruses, CHC-1 and CHV-2 have been isolated from red deer (Vanderplasschen et al., 1993); the former was associated with conjunctivitis in farmed red deer calves in Scotland (Nettleton et al., 1986). Rangiferine Herpesvirus-1 was isolated from a reindeer (Ek-Kommonen et al., 1986). CHV-1 and RHV-1 are related to Bovine herpesvirus-1, the cause of infectious bovine rhinotracheitis (Lyaku et al., 1992). A herpesvirus related antigenically to Equine Herpesvirus-1 was isolated from fallow deer in Alberta (Kinyili and Thorsen, 1979). Only CHV-1 has been associated with disease in farmed deer, and no herpesviruses have been firmly associated with disease in wild deer. However, antibodies that react with BHV-1 have been detected in Quebec caribou (Elazhary et al., 1981), and in black-tailed deer and white-tailed deer in the USA (Ingebrigtsen et al., 1986; Haigh and Hudson, 1993), and in white-tailed deer on Anticosti Island, where the herpesvirus was circumstantially associated with unusual mortality that occurred in deer in 1985 (Sadi et al., 1991).

Although these herpesviruses cross-react, indicating that they are antigenically related, they are distinct, and may very well not cross-infect significantly between hosts (Reid et al., 1986).

Status in Canada/Ontario

The status in Ontario is unknown. Herpesvirus has been isolated from fallow deer in Alberta, and antibody to an "herpesvirus has been demonstrated in parts of the USA and Canada.

Species: Fallow deer, red deer have been affected with (CHV-1, 2), and an uncharacterised herpesvirus has affected white-tailed deer and mule deer.

Probability of Entry/Transmission/Endemicity

Overall, Low. There is high probability of entry, because these viruses may be latent, and serology can be difficult. But a herpesvirus is circumstantially already present in white-tailed deer in North America. The transmission of herpesvirus requires close contact and the likelihood of establishment across host species barriers is low. In these circumstances, the incremental likelihood of transmission from farmed deer is likely low.

Low-to-moderate: Clinical disease can be severe with related herpesviruses in housed cattle. In deer, so far, the disease, known to be due to herpesviruses has been mild to non-existent. The association with high mortality on Anticosti Island is retrospective and speculative, but cannot be discounted.

Control/Mitigation

The best means of control is to ensure deer are contained on-farm.

Malignant Catarrhal Fever (MFC)

MFC is caused by a cell-associated (herpesvirus, either Alcelaphine Herpesvirus-1 transmitted from wildebeest (an issue in zoos), or Ovine Herpesvirus-2 (OHV-2) transmitted from domestic sheep. Until recently, tests were not available to detect carrier sheep or wildebeest, and they are still not routine (Baxter et al., 1993; Tham et al., 1994). The hosts of origin (wildebeest, sheep) do not develop disease, but the carrier state is widespread and common among them (Li et al., 1994, 1995).

Disease occurs in cattle, bison, and most species of cervids. Transmission is by exposure of the susceptible species to the carrier host, usually by close contact, since the virus is not persistent in the environment.

There is little, if any, horizontal transmission of disease among individuals of the susceptible species, despite the fact that they show severe signs (ocular; nervous; orocutaneous, respiratory, gastrointestinal mucosal ulceration). They are considered "dead end" hosts from the standpoint of disease transmission. Virtually all deer which develop clinical MCF go on to die (Haigh and Hudson, 1993).

Status in Canada/Ontario

Endemic infection with OHV-2 in sheep.

Species: Virtually all cervid species are susceptible to MCF, except fallow deer, which seem refractory to the disease. Sika deer, white-tailed deer, and red deer are highly susceptible; elk and perhaps mule deer seem less-so, but still may get the disease. Moose are also susceptible.

Probability of Entry/Transmission/Endemicity

Negligible: OHV-2 is present in sheep in Ontario, and farmed deer. Cattle and bison do become infected, but deer are dead end hosts, and endemic infection will not establish in farmed or wild deer.

High in captive deer, in which outbreaks can be devastating (Brown and Bloss, 1992); low in wild deer, in which it has rarely been reported (Jessup, 1985).

The risk to the wild population, from farmed deer is negligible, since deer-to-deer transmission is not significant.

Control/Mitigation

Prevent exposure of deer to sheep.

Parapoxviruses of Deer

Parapoxviruses usually cause mild transient infections in their native host, but can cause severe disease in unnatural hosts; however, the capacity to cross-infect, and the reaction in the unnatural host, are unpredictable. No parapox infections have been recognised in native deer in North America, and the only cervid in which a parapox infection is described is the red deer. In red deer, lesions of the skin and velvet antler were associated with cutaneous trauma due to thistles in paddocks (Haigh and Hudson, 1993). The overall impact of the disease was mild.

Status in Canada/Ontario

Unknown; red deer have been imported to Canada, but to Barker's knowledge, no disease compatible with parapox infection has occurred in that species here. A single case of uncharacterised parapox infection has occurred in an elk in western Canada (Haigh and Hudson, 1993), and there may be undescribed parapox viruses in elk and other deer. However, if present, they would seem to be uncommon.

Species: Red deer and presumably elk can be infected. Infectivity to other deer is possible but unproven.

Probability of Entry/Transmission/Endemicity

The virus may be spread by clinically-infected animals, which would likely get picked up in pre-shipment quarantine. However, incubating animals would not be detected, unless they got sick in quarantine here. The virus is also transmitted environmentally, and contact with an infected animal is not required. The capacity to cross-infect to other deer species is unknown, but other parapoxviruses readily cross species barriers.

Fungal Diseases

Anaplasmosis

Anaplasmosis is caused by the vector borne rickettsial organism Anaplasma marginale. It causes subclinical infection in an array of wild ungulates in the United States, and is capable of causing hemolytic disease in cattle (Radostits et al., 1994). Certain species of ticks act as biological vectors while tabanid (horse) flies act as mechanical vectors.

Status in Canada/Ontario —Exotic

Subclinical in wild ungulates, including certain species of deer (Haigh and Hudson, 1993); cattle and possibly mule deer (Haigh and Hudson, 1993) are at risk of illness.

Entry/Transmission/Endemicity

Low: Cattle and cervids are tested serologically prior to entry, and reactors are rejected. Entry from United States related to fraudulent documentation of imported cattle; re-use of needles contaminated with infected blood; or unexplained (?vector movement). Farmed cervids represent little additional risk beyond that posed by imports of cattle, and movements of free-ranging wild ungulates.

The capacity of the disease to become endemic is related to the availability of effective vector locally. It is more likely in western Canada where Dermacentor andersoni, a known vector, is present. When introduced into Canada with cattle in the past (Manitoba-1968; Quebec-1979; Saskatchewan-1983; Ontario-1996), it was successfully eradicated with attention to cattle only (Salsberg, pers. com., 1997), suggesting that it did not become established in local vector populations and wildlife.

Control/Mitigation

CFIA import control/testing and the eradication or re-export of carrier cattle detected after entry.

Parasitic Diseases

Ectoparasites

The principal ectoparasites (external parasites) of concern on deer are mites, especially Psoroptes. sp., and ticks, especially the winter tick Dermacentor albipictus and the black-legged tick Ixodes scapularis.

Psoroptes causes scabies on deer, including elk (Colwell and Dunlap, 1975; Samuel et al., 1991) and white-tailed deer (Bubenik, 1989; Garris et al., 1991), in which it may also cause otitis (Rollor et al., 1978), and it also infects mule deer (Roberts et al., 1970). Psoroptic scabies does not seem to be a clinical problem in red deer and fallow deer, but Sarcoptes mites have been recorded from red deer in Europe (Haigh and Hudson, 1993).

Dermacentor albipictus causes severe alopecia in moose, and does infect elk and white-tailed deer (Haigh and Hudson, 1993). Ixodes scapularis is the vector of Lyme borreliosis. It is endemic in parts of the northeastern and upper midwest USA, but is known to be endemic in Canada at only two localities in southern Ontario, Long Point peninsula (Barker et al., 1992), and Point Pelee National Park (Barker, unpublished).

Status in Canada/Ontario

Psoroptes, Dermacentor albipictus and Ixodes scapularis endemic on deer in Ontario, though Dermacentor albipictus is mainly associated with moose, and Ixodes scapularis is limited in distribution.

Species: Particularly white-tailed deer and elk, though any species of deer, as well as other medium-sized to large mammals, such as dogs, may be hosts for Ixodes scapularis.

Probability of Entry/Transmission/Endemicity

High, if animals come from endemic areas at a time of year when infestation is present (if seasonal). Establishment of endemicity in a new locality is dependent on local environment and climate. There is a high probability of establishment for Psoroptes, Dermacentor in Ontario and regionally variable for Ixodes scapularis (Lindsay et al., 1995). It is probably a greater issue with translocation of wild animals into or within the province, than with farmed deer.

There is no incremental harm, unless introduced into currently non-endemic locality and able to establish; then the degree of harm would be low to moderate. In endemic areas, deer farms pose no incremental risk. The impact of Ixodes scapularis is on people, not directly on wildlife.

Control/Mitigation

It is difficult to prevent introduction of ectoparasites by inspection or treatment with parasiticides. Animals should be moved at times of year when not infested with seasonal parasites (ticks). Confinement will limit contact transmission of mites somewhat; but confinement is unlikely to be effective with ticks.

Elaeophoriasis

The nematode Elaeophora schneideri, which inhabits arteries in the head and neck, infects mule deer with little effect, but causes problems with mastication in white-tailed deer; blindness, brain damage and gangrene of the tissues of the head in moose and elk; and less severe effects in sika deer and sheep and goats (Haigh and Hudson, 1993). The normal host in the western United States is the mule deer, and white-tailed deer are usually not infected. In the southeastern USA, white-tailed deer are the normal host. Elaeophora uses certain species of tabanids (horse flies) as vectors.

Status in Canada/Ontario

Present in British Columbia, never known in Ontario.

Likely all species of farmed deer, plus moose.

Probability of Entry/Transmission/Endemicity

Low to Negligible: The species of tabanid flies which are suitable vectors for this parasite do not seem to be present in Ontario, based on the natural absence of this worm from wild populations of white-tailed deer. Hence, even if an infected animal were imported, it would likely not transmit and establish.

Control/Mitigation

Not necessary under current circumstances.

Elaphostrongylus Cervi

This protostrongylid nematode, though it lives at sites distant from the lungs, produces eggs which reach the lungs via the circulatory system. The eggs hatch in the lungs and the first-stage larvae move up the trachea, and are swallowed, to be passed in feces (Mason, 1989). They use molluscs (snails or slugs) as intermediate hosts. Suitable molluscs are present and widespread in Canada (Gajadhar and Tessaro, 1995). Infectious larvae in molluscs accidentally ingested by deer, migrate from the gut to the spinal cord and brain, then, in most cases, to intermuscular tissues, where they mature. During their migration in the central nervous system, these worms can cause damage which may result in clinical disease.

Elaphostrongylus cervi is endemic in red deer populations in western Europe and New Zealand (Mason et al., 1976), though not in fallow deer (Mason, 1989). It is unknown in native species of cervids in North America, though elk in New Zealand have become infected spontaneously (Mason and McCallum, 1976). A related species, originally identified as E. cervi (Lankester and Northcott, 1979), but now considered to be E. rangiferi (Carreno and Lankester, 1993), a parasite of reindeer in Scandinavia (Bye and Halvorsen, 1984), probably was introduced by the translocation of European reindeer into Newfoundland, where it causes disease in caribou and moose (Lankester and Fong, 1989).

Elaphostrongylus alces is found in moose in Scandinavia (Steen et al., 1989). These parasites, though they do cross-infect hosts, seem to be distinct species (Steen et al., 1997), and separate from E. cervi, with which they were once lumped (Mason, 1995).

E. cervi has very low pathogenicity in red deer, causing usually minor lesions (Sutherland, 1976) detected at low frequency at meat inspection, and uncommonly in farmed animals (Mason and Gordon, 1994). In mule deer it will produce patent infections (animals pass larvae), but it causes significant central nervous system disease, resulting in ataxia and other neurologic deficits (Gajadhar and Tessaro, 1995) which may be fatal, or render the animal more prone to predation. White-tailed deer do not develop patent infections following experimental inoculation with E. cervi, and developing worms seem to be overcome by the host during their migration, without producing disease (A. Gajadhar, personal communication, 1998). Both E. rangiferi and E. alces also seem capable of causing disease in some other species of cervids, in addition to their natural host (Lankester and Fong, 1989).

In 1991 presumptive infection with Elaphostrongylus cervi was detected in several consignments of quarantined red deer imported to Canada from New Zealand, all of which were slaughtered (Gajadhar et al., 1994; deWith et al., 1998). Since the Baermann technique for detection of larvae in feces is insufficiently sensitive to reliably detect larvae in all infected animals importations of red deer and fallow deer from New Zealand (or elsewhere) that are not known to be free of E. cervi were halted in 1991 by Agriculture Canada, so as not to further imperil Canadian wildlife populations. The burden of proof with respect to freedom from infection is on the exporting country, and deer have not been imported into Canada from New Zealand since that time.

Of over 92,000 deer (?all species) examined in quarantine in New Zealand before export to Canada and Australia up to the end of 1990,

0.28% were detected shedding E. cervi larvae (P. Mason, Meeting on Elaphostrongylus cervi Risk Management for the Importation of Deer, Agriculture Canada, 1991). Among about 8,000 red deer in quarantine in Canada examined by the Baermann technique, about 0.1% were found to be infected (Meeting on Elaphostrongylus cervi Risk Management for the Importation of Deer, Agriculture Canada, 1991), though since all affected animals were detected in 1991, after an increase in sensitivity of the testing protocol, up to about 1% of animals may have been infected (de With et al, 1998). Probably no more than about 80 E. cervi-infected deer entered Canada, and of those, one can assume that about 20% were slaughtered without being released from quarantine (all those detected, and any undetected infected cohorts in the same consignments). The prevalence of infection with E. cervi among animals released from quarantine must have been very small (<~1%), if it was present at all.

Some red deer destined for slaughter from a consignment detected with E. cervi in quarantine, escaped as they were unloaded at an abattoir in southern Ontario; however, all were subsequently accounted for. Agriculture Canada took the position that, as of November 28, 1991, "Elaphostrongylus cervi has not been detected in continental Canada and that we can reasonably assume that it is not present." To our knowledge, this position has not been tested by seeking this parasite in red deer populations on farms in Ontario. Elaphostrongylus cervi infection would be unlikely to be detected in red deer unless sought specifically. Though the Baermann technique is relatively insensitive on an individual animal basis, it would likely detect established infections at the herd level if the prevalence of infection in individuals in herds of over 50-100 animals were substantial (>5-10%).

CFIA is currently developing an ELISA test capable of detecting animals with E. cervi early in the course of infection. This test is very promising, but, pending technical refinements and validation, is likely several years away from field application (A. Gajadhar, personal communication, 1998). No ELISA test has 100% sensitivity; however, such a test could be used effectively to detect infected herds, if not all infected individuals. Over a course of several herd tests at intervals, herds of susceptible species might be certified free of infection. Indeed, the same might be accomplished in herds of sufficient size now, using the Baermann technique, with repeated sampling, though infections with Parelaphostrongylus tenuis might yield false positive results. Infected herds would likely persist, due to the difficulty of eliminating infected molluscs from a premises. Since E. cervi is not amenable to successful therapy using anthelmintics currently available, potentially infected deer could not be placed in secure quarantine, treated, and safely moved to uninfected premises.

Other Elaphostrongylus *spp. are not reviewed since their hosts are not permitted to be farmed in Ontario.*

Status in Canada/Ontario

Not present in western Canada (west of Ontario, since red deer are not permitted); officially not present in eastern Canada/Ontario, but a slight possibility exists that it escaped quarantine.

Red deer from New Zealand and their descendants are potential hosts for endemic infection in Ontario. Elk are a susceptible farmed and indigenous wild species. Mule deer are a susceptible farmed species; while white-tailed deer and fallow deer are apparently insusceptible.

Probability of Entry/Transmission/Endemicity

Moderate, based on the possibility that it may have escaped quarantine, and could be endemic in red deer. Apparently there is no possibility of the establishing of Elaphostrongylus spp. in wild white-tailed deer. There is a possibility of the transfer of Elaphostrongylus spp. to elk, were infected deer to be farmed in an area where elk are established.

Low to moderate; potential impact on elk rather than white-tailed deer, even if difficult to eradicate from red deer. This is a potential issue in interprovincial trade if established, or status unknown.

Control/Mitigation

Control measures include CFIA import controls, possible testing and herd certification, zoning of deer farming away from elk range and the identification and confinement of farmed deer.

Gastrointestinal nematodes

Gastrointestinal nematodes, predominantly Trichostrongyloidea, are common in all ruminants, including deer. Infections typically involve a complex of species of worms, but are usually dominated by one. Those found in deer are usually species related, but not identical, to those in domestic ruminants, and even when they are the same species, they seem to be host-adapted. Parasites exotic to the new world certainly have been imported with their hosts to North and South America (Suarez at al., 1991; Rickard et al., 1993). Parasites of deer non-indigenous to Ontario may not transmit effectively to indigenous species of deer, although cross-infection by some species clearly can occur from white-tailed deer to exotics in areas of sympatry (Richardson and Demarais, 1992).

Worms parasitizing the abomasum (true stomach), belonging to the genus Ostertagia or its relatives, are pathogenic in fallow deer, red deer and wapiti, causing diarrhea and weight loss (Mylrea et al., 1991; Haigh and Hudson, 1993; Connan, 1996), as do their relatives in sheep and cattle. Related worms are found in wild white-tailed deer in Ontario (Baker and Anderson, 1975). Haemonchus species cause anemia in white-tailed deer in the southeastern United States, where, under warm, humid conditions, parasite burdens can be heavy. Under conditions prevailing there, worm burdens are host-density dependent, and have been used as a management tool in measuring deer population density in relation to habitat quality (Prestwood and Pursglove, 1981).

Status in Canada/Ontario

Endemic in farmed and wild deer, but species and host range of parasites may differ.

All farmed cervids and all wild cervids

Probability of Entry/Transmission/Endemicity

The probability of entry is high, but likelihood of establishment across host species barriers is moderate-to-low.

Low; probability of overt disease slight.

Control/Mitigation

Control measures include ensuring the deer are properly contained on the farm premises and limiting environmental contamination (runoff).

Lungworms

Lungworms of the genus Dictyocaulus occur in all species of deer and seem to be particularly pathogenic in red deer and elk. Most lungworms of deer (red deer, elk, white-tailed and black-tailed deer, reindeer and caribou, and moose) on morphologic grounds are termed D. viviparus (Anderson and Prestwood, 1981), which is the lungworm of cattle. Transmission is direct (no intermediate host). Cross infections do occur, but cross-infectivity of these worms among hosts in some cases seems to be incomplete (Anderson and Prestwood, 1981). When it has been attempted (ie. infectivity is best or pathogenicity is greatest in the host of origin, compared with the alternative host). There is argument about the nomenclature of the Dictyocaulus species of fallow deer in Europe, which seems to be a distinct species D. eckerti (Epe et al., 1997).

Dictyocaulus is an important pathogen of red deer, elk and fallow deer in captivity, including in Ontario (Appendix 6; Barker unpublished). Heavy infections can occur in wild deer, especially elk in the northern Pacific coast region (Haigh and Hudson, 1993) and white-tailed deer in the southeastern United States (Anderson and Prestwood, 1981). In Ontario, it seems only to be a minor parasite of wild deer, although it was implicated as a contributory agent in multifactorial winter deaths of deer in NewYork (Anderson and Prestwood, 1981).

Common Joint Diseases of Horses

Overview of Joints and Diseases

The junction between any two bones is known as an articulation or a joint. There are several types of joints. Some are fixed or practically immovable, such as those found between the skull bones. Others are freely movable and have articular cartilage and joint capsules.

The articular cartilage covers the ends of the bones and reduces friction between bones. The joint capsule surrounds the joint and consists of a tough, outer coat and a thin inner layer which lines it. This inner layer is termed the synovial layer and it produces a fluid known as the synovial fluid. This fluid resembles egg white in consistency and lubricates the joint when the bones move against one another.

Parts of the outer layer of some joint capsules are thickened to form ligaments. Ligaments connect bone to bone while tendons connect muscle to bone.

Arthritis is an inflammation of a joint involving the bones, the articular cartilages, ligaments and joint capsules. In an infected or irritated joint the amount of fluid increases and produces swelling. Bacteria may enter the joint through a wound of the joint capsule resulting in damage to the bones and cartilages. The joint may then become immovable.

To treat this condition the affected joint is rested. Medication is used to counteract the inflammation. If the arthritis is severe, immobilisation and resting of the joint is continued for 4 to 6 weeks. The outcome is usual favourable if bone damage or new bone growth has not occurred.

An injury to a ligament is defined as a sprain. Some ligaments hold bones firmly together and allow very little movement; others allow considerable movement. If an abnormal stress or movement is placed upon a joint such as overextension of a joint, the ligament may be torn. The amount of injury depends upon how much force is placed upon the ligament. If the ligament is torn completely away from its attachments to a bone, recovery is difficult. Adequate rest is necessary in hope that the torn ligament may repair itself.

Joint mice are pieces of bone or cartilage found within the joint cavity and may be the result of a fracture. These produce pain when lodged between the articular surfaces and may also produce arthritis. Surgical removal is usually successful.

A "stifled" horse results from the "locking" of the patella (knee cap of man) in the stifle joint. Normally a horse stands for hours without tiring of the hindlimb musculature. This is due to the "locking" mechanism of the hindlimb. The "locking mechanism" consists of the loop formed by the junction of two patellar ligaments with the patella and the bony projection of the lower end of the femur (thigh bone).

The stifle joint is locked in an extended or straightened stiff position whenever the horse is unable to "unlock" the loop of ligaments from over the bony projection. Sometimes a slap on the croup will cause the horse to jump and "unlock" the stifle joint. Often his "locking" will reoccur. Whenever surgery is necessary to correct the condition, the medial patellar ligament is cut on the inside of the stifle joint in order to prevent further "locking".

Bone Spavin

Bone spavin is defined as an inflammation of one or more bones of the hock and most often causes an arthritic condition of the affected bones. In bone spavin the joint between the bones on the inside of the hock become immovable. Quick stops,such as those which occur during roping and other stresses, along with mineral deficiencies, may produce bone spavin. Horses with full, well-developed hocks tend to have less incidence of bone spavin than those with narrow, thin hocks. Bone spavin occurs on the inside of the hock (jack spavin). It may occur between the bones within the hock joint and cannot be seen or palpated (blind spavin). A large percentage of horses affected with blind spavin recover completely.

Jack spavin is usually a bony growth of variable size. The bony enlargement pushes out against a tendon that lies over the inside hock area. The cause of bony growth cannot be fully explained. When the hock is flexed or bent, pain is produced and as a result the hindlimb is not raised very high. Therefore, the horse drags his foot.

Treatment consists of alleviating as much pain as possible. By cutting the tendon veterinarians can remove one source of pain. However, the outlook for full recovery from jack spavin is usually not favourable even with surgery. The horse will probably be useable, but rest and time are needed for repair to occur.

Bog Spavin

There is no bony enlargement; swelling, heat and pain are most evident on the front surface of the hock.

The cause may be due to nutritional deficiencies, accidental injury to the hock joint or the hocks being too straight (hereditary). If the condition is caused by conformation or too straight hocks, it cannot be treated successfully. Veterinarians have many factors to consider in order to determine the cause and to advise the best treatment. Anti-inflammatory drugs may help bog spavin caused by nutritional deficiencies or injury. The drugs decrease inflammation and prevent swelling of the joint capsule. A bandage around the hock prevents excessive build-up of fluid and swelling. The horse is rested for 4 to 6 weeks. Adding vitamins and minerals to the diet may relieve bog spavin. Horses 6 months to 2 years of age are most often affected with bog spavin.

Ring Bone

This condition is characterised by new bone growth which occurs on the first, second or third phalanx (high or low ringbone). The phalanges are the three small bones extending from the fetlock to the hoof. Ringbone is more common on the forefeet than the hindfeet.

Ringbone is due to an inflammation of the tough fibrous layer which surrounds the bones. The inflammation may be caused by stresses which pull on ligaments attached to the bone. The new bone growth may lead to arthritis and stiffening of the joints between the fetlock and the pastern. If the tough, fibrous layer surrounding the bones is cut (such as in wire cuts), new bone growth may result. The new bone may grow into the joints between the phalanges and produce stiffening of the joints. In early ringbone, swelling and heat are present over the affected areas. To assure a complete diagnosis, it is necessary to take radiographs. Again the veterinarian has many factors to consider in advising the best treatment. If the joints are involved, chances for full recovery are poor. Immobilisation of the foot and a long period of rest are often necessary. Corrective shoeing is also advisable in some cases.

Animal Health Lab

The Animal Health unit of the Laboratory Services Division provides a full-service, fully accredited veterinary diagnostic laboratory that supports provincial animal disease diagnosis and surveillance. Scientists and technologists at the AHL link their expertise with University of Guelph personnel to provide a single source of laboratory service in animal health, encompassing food-producing animals (livestock and poultry), exotic and zoo animals, companion animals and avian and mammalian wildlife populations.

The Ontario Ministry of Agriculture, Food and Rural Affairs and the University of Guelph provide a critical mass of leading veterinary specialists and laboratory staff that contribute to achieving high quality and efficient testing.

The new Pathobiology/Animal Health Laboratory being built on the corner of Gordon Street and McGilvray Street in Guelph will further safeguard animal and human health in Ontario. More about AHL

Agriculture and Food Lab (AFL)

The Agriculture and Food Laboratory (AFL) unit of Laboratory Services Division at the University of Guelph has been delivering accurate results for clients in agriculture, food and beverage, corporate and research sectors for over 30 years. With strong alliances in industry, government and academic sectors, this lab provides excellence in food quality and safety testing in Ontario and across Canada.

The AFL provides OMAFRA with high quality, special purpose laboratory services in support of the agriculture and food sectors and rural communities. OMAFRA and the AFL work collaboratively on the annual development of project descriptions and sampling plans that will fulfill the needs of the AFL's many clients. More about AFL.

Chapter 5

Health Protection and Sanitation Strategies for Cattle

Livestock owners and industry personnel who support their farms are genuinely concerned with the health, wellbeing and productivity of Ontario's cattle. They recognise that disease outbreaks are preventable. They adopt health management practices to prevent the introduction and/or spread of diseases in Ontario's herds.

There are very sound economic reasons for disease prevention. Some herd owners spend thousands of dollars each year fighting disease outbreaks. There are many more costs associated with chronic diseases that may go unnoticed.

In addition to the costs of health care, valuable livestock and production are also lost. Animal welfare, pride in stockmanship and peace of mind are also major incentives to minimise disease occurrence. Some diseases can be spread through the air. These are difficult to prevent. However, good biosecurity, nutrition, early disease detection and overall health management will help minimise the impact of air-borne diseases.

This Factsheet describes management strategies to prevent the introduction of disease to a farm or control the spread of disease amongst animals within a farm. Although the Factsheet refers specifically to cattle, the general strategies are applicable to other farm livestock.

The management strategies that prevent the entry and spread of disease can also be called the "biosecurity plan" for the farm. Every farm should have a biosecurity plan as part of its overall health management strategy.

A section on the control of foreign animal diseases appears at the end of this Factsheet.

Prevent the Introduction of Disease

Management of New Arrivals

Contagious diseases are transmitted directly from an infected animal to an uninfected animal. This is the most common method of disease transmission amongst animals. There are four main strategies for managing the potential introduction of disease when adding animals to the farm.

Maintain a Closed Herd

The first method is not to purchase cattle. For practical reasons there are few truly closed herds in Ontario. Owners would have to strictly adhere to the following requirements:

- use home-grown replacements for maintaining and increasing herd size
- prevent fence-line contacts of their stock with other cattle
- use artificial insemination for breeding and not bring in bulls
- not exhibit at shows
- restrict visitors.

Isolate New Arrivals

Quarantine of incoming animals is ideal. In most herds, minimising contact with the rest of the herd may be the only practical method of isolation. To isolate new arrivals:

- use separate housing, feeding and birthing areas (ideal)
- use separate housing and feeding areas (acceptable)
- prevent contact with other animals (minimum acceptable)
- prevent manure movement from the isolation area to the rest of the herd
- isolate for 21-30 days
- observe and examine for early disease detection
- milk isolated cows last
- test for diseases prior to addition to the main herd.

Know the Source of Purchases and Use Laboratory Testing

Many owners take precautions when purchasing animals. They also use laboratory-testing programs to maintain minimal disease herds or disease-free herd status. To know the health status of herd additions:

- purchase pregnant or virgin heifers to minimise the risk of introducing mastitis
- determine the vaccination and health status of individuals and the herd of origin
- purchase from herds of known health status such as those certified under the Canada Health Accredited Herds program.

The 21-30 day isolation period is ideal for:

- bacterial culture of milk and
- blood testing for specific diseases.

Use Vaccines

Vaccines are commonly used to protect cattle against respiratory disease and abortion. For herd additions, these vaccines may be given during the 21 to 30-day isolation period. Bovine virus diarrhea (BVD) and infectious bovine rhinotracheitis (IBR) have been diagnosed in Ontario herds. Vaccination against these two diseases should be the cornerstone of every herd vaccination program. Consult your veterinarian for specific recommendations on these and other aspects of health management for livestock.

Prevent the Spread of Diseases

Management of Farm Traffic

Bacteria, viruses or other agents of disease are infectious when they are capable of causing infection in exposed animals. Farm visitors wearing boots or clothing freshly contaminated with infectious agents can spread diseases within a farm and among farms. Birds, rodents, pets, people, equipment and vehicles contaminated with manure (or other bodily excretions) are potential disease carriers.

Control Birds

Pigeons, sparrows, starlings and swallows are the most common birds found in and outside barns. They may carry infectious agents on their feet and within their digestive system. To control bird populations:

- plug small and large nesting holes and perches in your barn that are suitable for sparrows and starlings
- screen all openings in natural ventilation dairy barns
- seal off openings into silo roofs
- screen ledges used as nesting sites by pigeons.

Control Rats and Mice

A rat deposits 25,000 droppings and a mouse deposits 17,000 droppings in one year. Even a small population of these rodents may severely contaminate feed supplies. In addition, rodents carry disease agents on their feet and fur, and they destroy millions of dollars worth of feed, supplies and buildings each year. To control rats and mice:

- construct rodent-proof buildings
- eliminate safe hiding places and nesting sites
- remove food and water supplies
- destroy existing populations by poisoning, fumigating, or trapping.

Control People and Pets

People spread contaminated material directly on footwear, hands and clothing. To decrease the spread of contaminants:

- inform herd workers, visitors and truckers of your farm protection methods and insist upon co-operation
- discourage visitors from entering the housing and feeding areas
- post "Do Not Enter" signs with a telephone number for contacting you on livestock buildings and farm entrance gates
- discourage visitors from touching cattle and calves
- designate a specific visitor area to minimise contacts
- insist visitors wash their boots before entering and leaving
- supply rubber boots or plastic disposable boots and clean coveralls for visitors
- provide a footbath containing disinfectant
- insist workers wash their hands before milking cows and after working with sick animals
- insist workers wear protective plastic or rubber gloves for calving cows
- control the movement of dogs and cats between farms
- minimise the contact of dogs and cats with animals and feeding areas
- vaccinate farm dogs and cats for rabies and diseases common in your area

- wash farm clothing with detergents and bleach or washing soda.

Control Vehicles and Traffic Patterns on the Farm

Vehicles spread contaminated material on their tires, fenders and undercarriages. To decrease the spread of contaminants by vehicles:

- provide a separate laneway for use by the milk truck in accordance with the regulations of the Milk Act. This laneway must not be contaminated with manure
- provide "clean" routes for feed delivery vehicles-routes that are not contaminated by manure
- provide cattle with laneways that do not cross lanes used by milk trucks and feed delivery vehicles
- avoid sharing manure handling equipment with neighbours
- wash equipment to be shared with neighbours and insist on clean equipment coming onto your farm.

The most common means of contaminating feed or feeding areas is by on-farm equipment used for handling manure.

To decrease this risk:

- avoid using manure handling equipment for handling feeds, and if necessary wash before using for handling feed
- lay out feed storage and manure handling sites to avoid common traffic routes
- design and build barns where cows do not cross feeding alleys.

Control Feed and Feeding Equipment

Consider contaminated feeds (forages, pasture, grains and concentrates, water and waste milk), feeding equipment and systems when developing an on-farm biosecurity plan. The section on managing vehicles and farm traffic provides some basic information. The biosecurity of feeding should include plans to:

- purchase from suppliers with quality assurance and monitoring programs
- protect feeds from contamination through proper storage of chemicals, pesticides and medications
- protect feed from manure contamination
- establish storage facilities for feeds for various classes of livestock and systems to avoid errors in feeding practices

- harvest feeds at proper moisture contents and ensile them in suitable storage systems
- monitor water quality and assure clean delivery systems.

Clean Equipment

Disease can spread from animal to animal and farm to farm indirectly by small and large equipment. To reduce this method of spread:

- keep visiting vehicles out of areas accessible to livestock
- thoroughly wash and disinfect the inside, outside and tires of equipment shared with neighbours
- use a new disposable needle for each animal when administering treatments
- disinfect dehorners, hoof knives and trimmers after using on each animal
- use your own halters and clippers rather than borrowing them
- use separate shovels and forks for feeding and manure handling
- sanitize nursing bottles and buckets after each calf feeding
- maintain clean water troughs, water bowls, and feed mangers
- clean and sanitize equipment and materials used for handling deadstock.

Management of Groups and Housing

Young animals acquire infectious diseases through exposure with older infected or carrier animals. Housing and management systems, especially for dairy cattle, are constructed to minimise contact between young and older animals. In effect, the young are given time to develop immunity to diseases before joining the adults. The facilities also permit implementation of feeding and management practices to assure maximum growth, health and comfort. Dairy cattle owners implementing these strategies should:

- implement maternity-pen and newborn-calf management practices that prevent calves from ingesting manure.
- separate pre-weaned dairy calves from all other age groups
- house each milk-fed dairy calf in an individual pen or hutch
- place hutches away from dairy barn exhaust fans
- alternatively, house milk-fed calves in groups of less than eight calves

- house 4-8-month-old dairy calves in groups separately from older heifers
- house yearling and breeding age dairy heifers separately
- separate dry dairy cows from milking cows
- implement practices to prevent the spread of contagious mastitis (e.g. segregate cows with mastitis to the end of the milking order, sanitize milking equipment after milking a mastitic cow)
- separate replacement beef heifers from the cows
- move beef cows to a clean pasture, away from the wintering area, for calving
- organise chore routine to feed and milk isolated cattle after the main herd
- provide adequate pen, stall or bedded area per animal
- provide adequate feed bunk length and water trough access per animal.

Sanitation and Disinfection Management

Spread of disease is reduced when premises are clean and sanitary. In some cases, provincial legislation assures that minimum standards will be maintained. For example, the Milk Act (1987) regulates sanitation on dairy farms in Ontario. Several common management procedures assure adequate sanitation of farm premises.

Disposal of Dead Animals

Carcasses can be a hazard to people and other animals. They can contaminate soil, air and water and require special handling. To minimise property contamination and risk of spreading disease, owners should:

- dispose of dead animals within 48 hours of their death
- include all contaminated bedding, milk, manure or feed
- prevent scavenging by dogs, cats, birds, foxes, coyotes, wolves or bears
- wear protective clothing
- clean and disinfect the area that was occupied by the dead cattle.

Producers may choose on-farm disposal methods or have the dead animal picked up by a licensed collector.

On-farm disposal options under the Disposal of Dead Farm Animals Regulation [O. Reg 106/09] include:

- burial
- composting
- incineration
- disposal vessels
- anaerobic digestion (in some cases).

For burial, incineration or composting the Regulation describes minimum separation distances from a number of features which include:

- livestock housing facilities
- field drainage tiles
- residential and commercial lands
- surface water
- bedrock and aquifers
- wells (including municipal wells and floodplains).

The regulation also includes specific guidelines for each disposal option and limitations on the volume of deadstock disposed of for each option.

Producers also may transport their own deadstock to:

- common bins
- waste disposal sites approved under the Environmental Protection Act
- disposal facilities licensed under the Food Safety and Quality Act, 2001 (FSQA) [Regulation 105/09]
- a licensed veterinarian for post mortem.

Deadstock may be picked up by a collector licensed under the FSQA. Federal regulations apply to the transportation of dead cattle. Cattle carcasses or Specified Risk Materials (SRM) removed from a carcass must be dyed with a visible stripe. SRM are tissues that have been shown in infected cattle to contain concentrated levels of the bovine spongiform encephalopathy (BSE) agent. Collectors are responsible for applying the dye prior to removal of carcasses.

Producers transporting their deadstock or SRM to a receiver must follow guidelines in the FSQA regulations. To move dead cattle or SRM off-farm, producers must obtain a free 90-day permit from the Canadian Food Inspection Agency (CFIA). The process may involve an on-farm inspection by CFIA staff.

Cattle that die during transportation are considered to be SRM. The transporter requires a permit to bring the carcass back to the premises of origin or to a facility that is permitted by the CFIA to store, process or dispose of SRM.

CFIA has a comprehensive set of documents that outline the policy related to components that may not be added to feed (the enhanced feed ban).

Manage Manure and Control Flies

Infected animals often shed infectious agents in their feces, urine and other bodily fluids. The agents may contaminate feed, water and housing. To reduce the risk of spreading disease by manure:

- plan and install manure systems to prevent environmental contamination and comply with the Minimum Distance Separation II formula
- compost or store manure under conditions that destroy most disease-producing bacteria
- remove manure frequently from barns, yards and holding areas to prevent completion of life cycles by parasites and flies
- control the fly population by removing manure, using traps, baits or flypaper, using insecticides, using biological predators (wasps) or combinations of control measures
- store manure so it is inaccessible to cattle, especially young stock
- protect young stock from exposure to manure piles
- assure clean teats and udders for nursing calves by using clean calving areas and bedding packs with clean straw or shavings.

Manage Maternity, Dick and Calf Pens

Exposure of freshening cattle and calves to infectious agents is reduced by carefully managing maternity and sick pens. For disease control:

- use maternity pens only for freshening cattle
- use sick pens only for sick cattle
- prevent animal-to-animal contact between sick pens and maternity pens

- clean all manure from the pens after use
- disinfect the walls and floors after use
- allow the pens to dry after disinfection
- bed the pens well before the next animal enters
- if applicable, move cows and heifers to clean, dry pastures or paddocks for calving.

Use Disinfectants

Information about disinfectants is available on the product label or from farm supply dealers, veterinarians, the Canadian Animal Health Institute and the product manufacturers.

The Canadian Compendium of Veterinary Products, 2009, 11th Edition, contains the monographs of many common disinfectants. The indications for use, special properties, advantages, cautions and directions are described for each product. Your veterinarian should have a copy of this book in his/her veterinary clinic.

Familiarize yourself with the product information contained on the product label or package insert before making a selection. For a particular application, determine if a product:

- has activity against bacteria, fungi or viruses
- is active in organic debris (manure)
- is effective in hard water
- has decreased or enhanced activity in heat
- has residual activity for a period of time after application
- is compatible with soaps
- is caustic or has irritating fumes
- can be used on feeding equipment
- can be disposed of in accordance with provincial regulations and
- is appropriate for the intended use.

Several disinfectants for stables, housing and footbaths for visitors are shown in Table. These were obtained from the Compendium of Veterinary Products and are listed as examples, not endorsement. Other products may be available. Use the product information brochure included with the product to determine if the disinfectant meets the criteria for your application.

Disinfectants fall into six major categories: chlorhexidine, formaldehyde/glutaraldehyde, iodine complex, isopropanol, phenolic, or quarternary ammonium disinfectants. Several disinfectants fall into the other category not included in those mentioned above.

Foreign Animal Disease

For more than 50 years, Canada has successfully used border and import restrictions to prevent the entry of foreign animal disease (FAD). Ontario's livestock producers support these actions and supplement them with some common sense on-farm strategies.

Border Control

Canada prevents the introduction of FAD by strict border controls. The Canadian Food Inspection Agency and Customs Canada continue to:

- assess the risk of specific products that other countries want to import
- assess the animal health system in other countries
- ban the importation of ruminant (and some other) animals and their products
- ban the importation of used farm equipment
- use "sniffer" beagles to find food products carried by passengers
- seize and destroy foodstuffs and other illegal imports
- question passengers and inspect their baggage
- use disinfectants for passengers' shoes
- conduct specific tests and inspections of animals entering Canada.

On-Farm Control

Ontario's livestock producers prevent the introduction of FAD by common sense and practical farm-gate strategies.

For example, food and mouth disease (FMD) virus is easily killed by common procedures for cleaning or washing clothes-dry cleaning, bleach or washing soda. Experiments carried out 30 years ago showed that people examining the head area of clinically affected pigs harboured the FMD virus in their nasal cavity for less than two days. In these trials, infection of FMD was transmitted by snorting and coughing into the noses of steers within 30 minutes after examining the affected pigs. Presumably, the concept of a "stand-down period" after exposure to FMD virus came from these experiments. This confirms that persons who have been working with FMD animals must stay away from healthy animals for more than two days.

To prevent the introduction of foreign animal diseases from infected animals on farms in countries with diseases, Ontario's producers should:

- ask foreign visitors about diseases in their country of origin
- ask foreign visitors about their attendance on farms in their country of origin
- ask about and check the cleanliness of shoes and clothes of visitors
- provide rubber boots and protective clothing
- provide plastic boots
- restrict visitors from their farm if the visitor has been on a farm with a contagious foreign animal disease within the previous five days.

In case of an outbreak of a foreign animal disease in Ontario, federal veterinarians may impose bans on cattle movements to prevent the spread of contagious diseases from animal to animal. There would also be other control actions to stop the disease from spreading.

Disinfectants for Boot Wash

- Phenolic disinfectants (Beaucoup and Multi Phenolic Disinfectant) are examples of this class of disinfectant. Follow the label directions for mixing with water.
- Iodophors. Iosan is an example. Generally, prepare the boot wash by mixing 2-4 oz/gal of water (60-120 mL/4.5 L).
- Hypochlorites. Clorox or other brands of bleach that contain 5.25% sodium hypochloride. Mix 2-4 oz/gal (60-120 cc/4.5 L) of water.
- Chlorhexidine. Hibitane Disinfectant (2% w/v). Mix 120 mL per 3.8 L water.
- Sulfates. Virkon is an example. The common dilution rate for Virkon is 1% weight/volume. Mix a 50-gm packet in 5 L water.

Organic material (dirt and manure) inactivates many disinfectants. Therefore, clean your boots with a brush and water, removing all dirt and manure so that the disinfectant will sanitize the boots. Hypochlorites and iodophors will cause deterioration of rubber boots if left in contact. Prolong boot life by rinsing them with clear water after thoroughly disinfecting.

Conclusion

The work of disease prevention is never finished. Owners have the ultimate responsibility for herd protection. Visitors must respect biosecurity protocols put in place by livestock owners. Savvy livestock owners implement biosecurity strategies to prevent the introduction of disease to their herds and also to prevent the spread of diseases already present. To protect their herds, owners commonly:

- manage new arrivals
- manage and control farm traffic
- manage groups of animals and their housing
- sanitize and disinfect
- impose "stand-down periods" for visitors from foreign countries.

Review strategies for health protection and sanitation management of your herd using the lists above. Consult a veterinarian regarding which biosecurity strategies to use in your herd health program. Implement the appropriate strategies to insure health and comfort for your cattle. Make sure all workers and visitors are aware of their role in safeguarding the health of the herd.

For foreign animal diseases, border controls are a major part of the national biosecurity line of defence. On-farm biosecurity is an equally important line of defence. Together these steps minimise the entry and impact of diseases on your farm and in Canada.

Bioterrorism Involving Livestock

In light of the recent events in North America, governments and the public have a heightened awareness and concern about the possibility of bioterrorism involving agriculture, including livestock. This alert is not meant to cause panic or overstate the obvious. However, veterinarians and livestock owners may be the first to diagnose the early cases of a bioterrorist act in agriculture, as livestock can be sentinels of such an exposure. At the very least this note provides further points of contact for more information.

The Centres for Disease Control and Prevention in the United States has produced a list of the most likely biological agents to be used in an act of bioterrorism. Many of these are pathogens shared by humans and animals, and some have agricultural significance. Other agents of concern include Foreign Animal Diseases and other reportable diseases (such as Foot and Mouth Disease, Avian Influenza). Although many of the pathogens listed as possible bioterrorism agents would cause localised or sporadic disease, some may have serious public health or trade implications.

Veterinarians should remain current and vigilant for clinical signs consistent with any reportable or foreign animal disease, as well as unusual patterns or clusters of disease from the agents listed below. The Animal Health Laboratory (University of Guelph) and other diagnostic laboratories across Canada have been notified to be on alert for the detection of such agents. Diseases or clusters that might point to an exposure consistent with an act of bioterrorism could include: unusual demographic patterns, multiple species involvement, concurrent animal/public health problems, and unusual clusters of strains or serotypes.

Disinfection in on-Farm Biosecurity Procedures

Since the appearance of foot-and-mouth disease (FMD) in Europe in early 2001, its possible introduction into the United States has caused many livestock owners serious concern, so much so that many are now looking more closely at their biosecurity plans or their efforts to keep the disease out of their herds. Extension veterinarians have received many calls regarding which disinfectants to use on shoes, boots, tires, or other equipment in order to kill the foot-and-mouth disease virus. A few important points about disinfection should be made before choosing a disinfectant for routine farm use.

First, most disinfectants won't work if the surface to be disinfected isn't clean before applying the disinfectant.

Steam and high-pressure washers can be very useful to clean porous surfaces. Organic materials such as soil, plant debris (like straw), milk, blood, pus, and manure often inactivate some disinfectants or protect germs from the disinfectant's active ingredients. Chlorine-based disinfectants are especially subject to this problem. Chlorine, the active ingredient in bleach, is relatively quickly inactivated by organic debris such as manure, and even milk, at the concentrations usually used on clean surfaces.

In addition, even "hard" water can reduce or destroy the activity of some disinfectants. Likewise, some disinfectant solutions are only active for a few days after mixing or preparing. Failure to make a fresh solution of disinfectant after it has been prepared longer than a few days, or after it has become visibly contaminated by organic material like manure, may result in using a product that doesn't really work. Even worse, it may give a false sense of security. It is true that sufficient concentration and contact time can overcome some of these problems with certain classes of disinfectants, but often increasing the concentration or contact time makes use of the product impractical, costly, or caustic.

Disinfectants also vary considerably in their activity against the assorted germs bacteria, viruses, fungi, and protozoa about which livestock producers are concerned.

For example, plain vinegar (4% acetic acid) will readily kill the foot-and-mouth disease virus, but it won't do much to *Mycobacterium paratuberculosis*, the cause of Johne's disease. Most commonly used disinfectants are not active against bacterial spores, the environmentally hardy life form taken by the germs that cause tetanus, blackleg, botulism, and anthrax. Yes, formaldehyde is effective against most spores, but it is not really a practical disinfectant and is now considered a potential cancer-causing compound.

It is important to select a disinfectant that will be active across a wide spectrum of germs under the conditions in which it will usually be used.

These conditions include hard water, contamination with organic material, and potential for toxicity or damage to environmental surfaces or skin and clothing. It is also important to keep solutions clean and freshly made as directed by the manufacturer.

Lastly, disinfectants must have sufficient contact time with the surfaces to which they are applied in order to allow them to kill the germs with which we are concerned.

Contact time needed varies with the product and the germ. A quick splash of a dirty boot in a foot bath is not likely to accomplish anything except to give a false sense of security.

The chart of disinfectants on the next page has recently been made available by the USDA for field use in a foot-and-mouth disease outbreak ** and is useful in examining some of the previously stated points.

As you can see from the above, common household bleach would be an effective disinfectant for the FMD virus, but the recommended concentration (3% sodium hypochlorite) is 60% of full strength as it comes from the bottle. This concentration would damage clothing, shoes, and rubber goods and is mildly corrosive to steel surfaces. It can be used on an infected premise for FMD, but probably wouldn't be a good choice as a general purpose disinfectant for equipment and foot baths. Vinegar will also kill the virus, but wouldn't be a good choice for general use because of its lack of effectiveness against many other important germs. Obviously, lye is too caustic for general use.

On most farms, disinfectants will be used in foot baths or for cleaning equipment and livestock premises. The most commonly used disinfectants fall into the following classes.

Quaternary ammonium. The older quaternary ammonium compounds (Roccal D^T^) are good for some situations and relatively clean surfaces. They will not be particularly effective against FMD or *M. paratuberculosis*, the cause of Johne's disease, and have markedly reduced activity in the presence of organic material. Some of the newer quaternary ammonium preparations have improved activity. Compounds in this class usually have some detergent action; however, they are usually inactivated in contact with many soaps or soap residues.

Phenol-based compounds. These compounds are coal-tar derivatives and often have a strong pine-tar odour. They usually turn milky when added to water and have good activity in hard water and in the presence of some organic material. They are considered active against many bacteria, viruses, and fungi, including the bacteria that cause tuberculosis and Johne's disease. They are not especially active against the FMD virus; however, they are good all-purpose disinfectants for farm use. Some examples of this class of disinfectants include One Stroke Environ^R^, Osyl^R^, and Amphyl^R^.

Hypochlorites. Chlorine compounds are good disinfectants on clean surfaces and have a broad spectrum of activity. They generally are more active in warm water. They can be somewhat irritating and can be harmful to clothing, rubber goods, and some metals. Some of the newer chlorine-based disinfectants are complex molecules that are less irritating and more effective than older ones such as bleach and Halazone^R^. Chlorine-based disinfectants are generally compatible with soaps but should never be mixed with acids. Their activity is strongly reduced by the presence of organic matter. Many chlorine solutions are unstable and need to be frequently replaced; read the label.

Iodophors. Iodine compounds have been used as antiseptics and disinfectants for many years. The iodophors are combinations of iodine and another molecule that makes them water-soluble. They are good disinfectants but are also not as effective in the presence of organic debris. Iodophors are generally less toxic than other disinfectants but can stain clothes and some surfaces. They are inactivated in the presence of some metals and by sunlight. They should not be mixed with quaternary ammonium disinfectants as they will be inactivated. Some examples of this class are Betadine^{R} and Weladol^{R}.

Newer compounds. New disinfectants are being introduced regularly. Some of these are oxidising agents. Virkon S^{R} is a peroxygen molecule/organic acid/surfactant combination (surfactants reduce surface tension to help water-based compounds penetrate). It appears to have a wide spectrum of activity against many kinds of germs (including the FMD virus). It is relatively stable in the presence of some organic material. It has a pH of around 2.6, when mixed as directed, but is labelled as nonirritating to skin. It is advertised as useful on many kinds of equipment, including saddles, brushes, buckets, etc. Another compound, based on peroxyacetic acid, is Oxy-Sept 333^{R}. It is now EPA-approved for foot-and-mouth disease virus and is reportedly active against a broad spectrum of germs.

Remember, disinfectants are not to be applied to animals directly, unless labelled for such use, and you should consult the label to make sure there are no warnings against using them around feeders and in animal quarters. A general recommendation is to rinse disinfectants off after the appropriate amount of contact time if animals will have contact with the disinfected surfaces. Label directions should be strictly followed, and different classes of disinfectants should not be mixed.

In the event of a foreign animal disease outbreak, such as FMD, the type of disinfectant and procedures used in the cleanup of infected farms and for routine prevention activities will be selected by regulatory officials. For routine use in biosecurity programs at the farm level, producers should consider the major risks they are concerned about, consider the type of surface they wish to disinfect, the conditions under which the disinfectant will be used, and then select a disinfectant that best suits their needs. Information about activity in hard water or in the presence of organic debris, contact time needed, what germs are reliably killed, human use and environmental concerns, and other details are usually on the label or can be obtained from the company. Web sites are often good sources of information about individual products. Above all, producers should remember that disinfection is just one aspect of their biosecurity program.

Infectious Laryngotracheitis

A clinical case of Infectious Laryngotracheitis (ILT) has been confirmed in a poultry flock in Oxford County. The case was diagnosed on December 11 based on samples submitted to the Animal Health

Laboratory at the University of Guelph. OMAFRA is working with the industry and the producer's veterinarian to reduce the risk of ILT spreading to other farms.

Producers are instructed to heighten biosecurity. The service industries, as well as provincially and federally licensed processing plants, are also advised to enhance their biosecurity procedures.

ILT is an acute respiratory disease caused by a herpes virus that can lead to devastating losses in the broiler and layer industries. The disease is most frequently associated with chickens, but can also cause disease in related birds such as pheasants and peafowl. Ontario has experienced ILT outbreaks in the past. The ILT virus does not cause infection in humans.

The mortality rate in affected flocks is usually low, although it can sometimes be more than 20%. Persistent shedding from recovered birds can prolong infection in a flock for a long period of time. The disease is normally characterised by gasping, neck extension, watery eyes (conjunctivitis), swollen sinuses and persistent nasal discharge. In severe cases, violent coughing may be observed, with blood evident in the trachea.

ILT spreads relatively slowly through a flock within 2-4 weeks. The disease is usually spread by people, vehicles or equipment contaminated from an infected farm. Producers must be particularly careful with respect to the disposal of dead birds and manure, as the virus can be spread by these routes. Infected farms are advised to partially compost manure in the barn for at least 3 days prior to removal for complete composting on premises.

Biosecurity is the most important means of prevention. The improper use of vaccines can result in clinical infection and further spread of the disease. Producers should consult their veterinarian to determine the appropriate biosecurity procedures for their operation.

Avian Influenza

Avian influenza (AI) is a contagious viral infection that can affect several species of food producing birds as well as pet birds and wild birds. AI viruses can be classified into two categories: low pathogenic (LPAI) and highly pathogenic (HPAI) forms, based on the severity of the illness caused in birds.

Avian influenza viruses, such as the highly pathogenic H5N1 virus present in Asia, may, on rare occasions, cause disease in humans. Transmission to humans has occurred through close contact with infected birds or heavily contaminated environments.

In Canada, highly pathogenic avian influenza is a reportable disease under the *Health of Animals Act*, and all cases must be reported to the Canadian Food Inspection Agency (CFIA).

Avian Influenza (AI)-What to Expect if Your Animals are Infected?

About Avian Influenza

AI is a viral disease of birds. There are many different strains of the AI virus, and most of these have little or no affect on bird health. However, two types—known as H5 and H7—can cause severe illness and death in affected flocks. The Canadian Food Inspection Agency (CFIA) initiates disease response actions when birds are suspected to be infected with H5 or H7 AI viruses or other AI viruses determined to be highly pathogenic.

AI viruses can be classified into two broad categories: low pathogenic (LPAI) and highly pathogenic (HPAI), based on the severity of the illness caused in chickens. HPAI causes the greatest number of deaths in birds.

In Canada, Highly Pathogenic AI (HPAI) is a "federally reportable disease". This means that producers, veterinarians and laboratories must notify the CFIA of all suspected or confirmed cases. Birds affected by AI can show a variety of symptoms, including:

- high mortality and sudden death
- decreased food consumption
- huddling, depression, closed eyes
- respiratory signs (coughing and sneezing)
- decreased egg production
- watery greenish diarrhea
- excessive thirst
- swollen wattles and combs.

Humans are rarely affected by AI, except in a limited number of cases when individuals were in close contact with infected birds. Nevertheless, public health authorities will take precautionary measures as warranted.

AI Disease Control

The CFIA takes immediate disease control actions in response to all situations where domestic birds are suspected of being infected with H5/H7 AI. While all disease response situations are different, the steps involved in an AI response normally include the following:

- movement restrictions, e.g., quarantines
- sample submission
- investigation
- destruction and disposal
- cleaning and disinfection
- compensation.

Quarantine

If you are a producer of a flock of birds that is suspected of being infected with H5/H7 or highly pathogenic AI, CFIA staff members will come to your farm to begin an investigation.

At that stage, a quarantine (also referred to as a Declaration of Infected Place) will be placed on your farm to control the potential spread of disease. You will be provided with documentation outlining the rules of the quarantine. Signs indicating that the property is a disease control area may also be provided. These signs must be posted at all entrances.

Under the quarantine, no birds, bird products (such as eggs) or bird by-products (such as manure) will be allowed to enter or leave your property without CFIA permission.

It is your responsibility to ensure people entering and exiting your property follow strict biosecurity measures, such as the cleaning and disinfection of footwear and vehicle tires. Other items being moved off the property will also need to be cleaned and disinfected under the direction of CFIA personnel.

While your property is under quarantine, you will have the following responsibilities:

- Request CFIA permission to move birds, bird products, bird by-products and poultry related equipment on or off the property.
- Ensure that footwear and vehicles leaving the property have been cleaned and disinfected.
- Apply strict biosecurity measures for yourself and any employees.
- Maintain fences and gates around the farm to control the movement of people on and off the premises.

- Where applicable, maintain fences and gates to areas housing birds—all birds should be housed indoors while the quarantine is in place.
- Report all sick and dying birds, and any that escape the farm.
- Implement vermin, feral animal, or wildlife control measures if warranted.
- Keep dogs, cats and other household pets confined.
- Inform all persons entering the farm of the quarantine.
- Limit on-farm visitors to essential services.

Investigation

The CFIA veterinarian will start the investigation by asking a series of questions about the health of your birds and the management practices you use. They will also attempt to answer any questions you may have.

To help CFIA staff in their investigation, you may be asked to provide the following information:

- flock records (e.g., mortality, production, feed and water intake)
- veterinary records and laboratory reports
- a detailed description of farm management practices
- records of purchase/sale of feed, poultry, etc.
- movement on and off the premises during the past 21 days, (e.g. feed trucks, power, gas)
- farm visitor logbooks
- a site map of the farm
- contact information for the farm veterinarian.

Any premises considered to be in significant contact with your farm will also be quarantined because of the potential for disease spread. An example of a significant contact farm would be if you shared farm equipment or recently exchanged birds with another bird owner.

Your cooperation and that of any other parties involved is critical to the success of the investigation.

Confirmation of AI

Testing to confirm if your birds are infected will be done as quickly as possible. Samples will be taken from the flock and sent to the nearest CFIA-approved laboratory. Testing to confirm the 'H' type can be completed within one or two days.

If H5 or H7 or highly pathogenic AI is confirmed, all birds on your property will be humanely destroyed. Poultry products, such as eggs, will be destroyed as they are considered to pose a risk of spreading the AI virus to other birds.

Flocks on other farms in the surrounding area will also be quarantined and tested.

If the particular virus present on your commercial farm is determined to be highly pathogenic, all the poultry on commercial operations within one kilometre of your commercial farm will also be pre-emptively destroyed.

If H5 or H7 is confirmed, local health authorities will be available to answer any human health concerns or questions that you may have.

Destruction and Disposal

All birds are humanely destroyed using internationally recognised methods. Carcasses are disposed of in accordance with provincial requirements. Common disposal methods include burial, composting or incineration. On-farm burial must comply with provincial and municipal waste management requirements. All destruction and disposal costs may be covered by the CFIA.

Compensation

Under the Health of Animals Act, the CFIA may compensate owners for animals and things ordered destroyed during disease response situations. Compensation awards are based on market value, up to the maximum amounts established by the regulations.

Cleaning and Disinfection

Farms on which infected birds lived must be cleaned and disinfected after all destruction and disposal activities have been completed. The CFIA conducts a site assessment with the owner to determine which areas require cleaning and disinfection. The cleaning and disinfection process includes:

- removing litter and manure
- wet cleaning and disinfecting hard surfaces and structures
- cleaning and disinfecting tools and equipment.

Cleaning and disinfecting costs are your responsibility.

Removal of Quarantine

Once cleaning and disinfection are complete on the premises, the CFIA evaluates the farm to determine when the quarantine may be removed. Normally, this occurs 21 days after the cleaning and disinfection final inspection and approval.

Following removal of the Declaration of Infected Place, you can introduce new birds to the farm in accordance with CFIA requirements.

Confidentiality

As directed by the Privacy Act and other federal statues, the CFIA is required to protect private information collected. Any information provided by you during a disease response situation is treated as confidential, unless otherwise indicated.

Questions or Concerns?

If you have any questions or concerns related to the CFIA's disease response activities, please contact:

How to Prevent and Detect Disease in Backyard Flocks and Pet Birds?

Diseases such as highly pathogenic avian influenza and velogenic Newcastle disease can cause serious illness and death in many bird species. Fortunately, you can protect your birds and keep them healthy.

Follow five basic rules in the day-to-day care of your birds to reduce the risks posed by harmful diseases.

Prevent Contact with Wild Birds and Other Animals

Wild birds and other animals such as mice can carry a range of disease-causing viruses, parasites and bacteria. Make sure that your birds and their food and water are kept away from wild animals. Promptly clean up spilled feed and litter, and keep feed in sealed containers to avoid attracting unwanted guests.

Clean, Clean and Clean

Viruses, parasites and bacteria can live in organic matter such as litter and soil. Eliminate the risk of disease spread by routinely and thoroughly cleaning barns, cages, egg trays, gardening tools, and water and feed containers. No equipment should be shared with or borrowed from other bird owners. Always clean your hands, clothing and footwear before and after handling birds. Promptly dispose of dead birds, litter and unused eggs.

Spot the Signs and Report Early

Bird owners are legally responsible to notify authorities of serious bird diseases such as avian influenza. Call a veterinarian or a local office of the Canadian Food Inspection Agency if you suspect your birds are sick.

Signs to look for include:

- lack of energy, movement or appetite;
- decreased egg production;
- swelling around the head, neck and eyes;
- coughing, gasping for air or sneezing;
- nervous signs, tremors or lack of coordination;
- diarrhea; or
- sudden death.

It is always better to be overcautious. Report any bird that you think may be sick. Early reporting can greatly limit the effect of a disease on the health of your birds.

Limit Exposure to Visitors

People can spread bird diseases, too. As a general rule, do not give visitors access to your birds. If someone must enter your property or handle your birds, make sure that their clothing, hands and footwear are clean and free of debris. Provide shoe or boot covers, or use a foot bath to prevent disease from entering or leaving your property. As well, the tires and wheel wells of any vehicles that have been around birds should be cleaned before entering your property.

Keep New Birds Separate when Entering Your Flock

Avoid introducing disease to your birds. New birds should be segregated and monitored for at least 30 days before entering your existing flock. Make sure that new birds come from reputable suppliers that have strict disease controls in place. Birds returning from shows or exhibits should also be segregated for at least two weeks

The Facts about Bird Flu

Avian Influenza (also known as "Bird Flu") continues to make headlines, sometimes causing confusion and anxiety among the general public. Is it safe to travel to Europe or Asia? Is it safe to eat poultry? Is it safe to go near wild birds?

Bird Flu, in its current form, is almost exclusively a disease of birds and does not pose a general threat to public health.

The reason that avian influenza and pandemic influenza have been linked together by some people is the potential for a virus usually found in animals to mutate and form a new virus that could easily infect humans, both directly and from one human to another. There is currently no human influenza pandemic in the world..

The following points may also help put Bird Flu into perspective.

- There are many different strains of Avian Influenza virus, commonly found in wild birds. Most cause no harm to birds or humans. The particular strain causing illness overseas is known as H5N1 (Asia).
- H5N1 (Asia) has not been detected in North America.
- Currently, H5N1 (Asia) does not cross easily from birds to humans. Almost all human cases to date resulted from direct contact with infected domestic birds or their droppings.
- There is no reason for the public to avoid eating properly cooked poultry and eggs.
- There is no evidence of cats infecting humans. A few cases of H5N1 (Asia) have been reported in domestic cats in Europe and Asia, but these were also caused by direct exposure to infected birds.
- The virus is likely being spread both by migrating wild birds and by the sometimes illegal movement of infected live poultry and on contaminated clothing and equipment. Wild birds may introduce the virus to a region or country, but poor biosecurity allows it to infect commercial poultry operations and spread to other farms.
- Because of migratory patterns, there is a chance that the virus will show up in wild birds this year in North America. The presence of the virus, however, does not necessarily mean that it will become widespread or that it will affect commercial poultry or humans. It certainly does not signal the start of a pandemic.

Notwithstanding all these facts, prevention and preparedness are appropriate at this time. The key to managing Bird Flu is controlling the disease in domestic poultry before it can become something more serious to humans as well as an economic disaster for the poultry industry. Another important step is minimising the contact, and possible mixing, among influenza viruses of birds, humans and other animals. Because of this, controlling the annual human flu virus through vaccination and good hygiene practices will also contribute to pandemic prevention, in addition to being a good public health measure.

What can be done to prevent the spread of Avian Influenza in Poultry?

- Governments are working with wildlife experts to detect the presence of Avian Influenza viruses in wild birds. Plans are in place for dealing with H5N1 if it is detected in wild or domestic birds in Canada.
- The commercial poultry industry is making biosecurity practices mandatory for its producers. It is important for all producers to follow these protocols routinely.
- There is currently no need to restrict or cancel poultry shows. However, bird owners should always observe proper biosecurity practices when attending any such event where birds from different sources are mixed.
- Bird owners, including hobbyists and those raising non-quota poultry, should follow these Biosecurity Basics to protect their birds from possible infection.

The 5 Biosecurity Basics for Bird Owners

- *Restrict visitor access.* People can bring diseases onto your farm, especially if they own or have been in contact with other birds. Contact with your birds should be restricted to those caring for them. It is a good idea to have separate clothing and footwear for use when dealing with your birds.
- *Prevent contact with wild birds and other animals.* Keep your birds in an enclosed or screened in area, and protect their food and water from contamination.
- *Don't bring disease home.* New additions or birds that have been at a fair or market should be isolated and observed for signs of disease for at least two weeks before joining the flock. Equipment such as cages should not be shared with other bird owners. Any shared equipment should be thoroughly washed and disinfected.
- *Keep it clean.* Routinely wash and disinfect cages, feed and water surfaces, boots and any equipment that comes in contact

with the birds or their droppings. Wash your hands thoroughly after dealing with the birds.

- *Recognise and report illness.* Early detection is critical in successfully dealing with a disease outbreak. It is better to be overcautious than too late. If your birds show signs of disease, such as depression, abnormal egg production or feed consumption, respiratory problems, diarrhea, or sudden death, call your local veterinarian or contact the Canadian Food Inspection Agency immediately.

Infectious Bursal Disease of Chickens (Gumboro Disease)

This syndrome was first recognised near Gumboro, Delaware in 1962. It was first recognised in this province in 1970. It appears to be almost universal in broiler-growing areas.

Cause

Gumboro Disease is caused by a small, hardy virus, which shares many characteristics of the reovirus group. The organism is resistant to a great range of temperature and pH, but is killed by most disinfectants (formalin, cresol, iodine, etc.). The virus is rapidly spread by direct contact between birds and can survive for extended periods of time on inanimate objects, contaminated feed, etc. It does not appear to spread through the air.

Clinical Signs

Whitish, watery or mucoid diarrhea may be evident in the flock, with very sticky litter and soiling of vent feathers. Many birds may be reluctant to move with a tendency to sit. There is listlessness, dehydration and some deaths, with poor feed conversions. Secondary disease conditions, such as E. Coli infection, Marek's disease, gangrenous dermatitis and inclusion body hepatitis may increase in incidence, and condemnation rates may be elevated. The mortality pattern may range from the normal acceptable levels to a total of 15%, but the usual rate is low.

Four days after the onset of clinical signs, the mortality peaks and returns to normal within a week. The number of affected birds in a flock (morbidity) is variable and can approach 100%. Sick birds do not die if management is good and stresses kept to a minimum. Apparently subclinical disease can occur and destroy the birds immune system without causing obvious illness in a flock until secondary diseases develop.

Disease

The bursa of Fabricius, which is the organ responsible for disease protection in young birds, is the main target for the virus. Normally, the bursa of Fabricius regresses by early maturity. Hence, infectious bursal disease is most important in birds up to 4 months of age, and most critical between 2 and 4 weeks of age. The virus destroys many of the cells in the bursa of Fabricius and the resultant inflammation causes the organ to enlarge in size. Fever may develop and may cause depression and dehydration. Kidney damage (nephrosis) may result from the dehydration.

Hemorrhagic lesions throughout the body on the breast and leg muscles are seen on occasion. The post-mortem findings include pale, swollen kidneys, abnormally large or small bursa, hemorrhagic muscle lesions and possibly damage to the spleen, thymus or cecal tonsils.

Diagnosis

Diagnosis is made on the flock history and postmortem examination, and confirmed by virus isolation and identification. Serology and fluorescent antibody techniques are now available and help identify the disease agent. Histopathology of the bursa can also lead to a diagnosis.

Treatment and Control

No known chemotherapeutic or antibiotic agent is effective in the treatment or control of infectious bursal disease. Drug therapy is often inadvisable in the presence of severe kidney damage. Electrolyte and/or multiple vitamin administration may be helpful in flocks where the disease is of relatively long standing and appetites poor. Good ventilation, warm temperatures and fresh water will help to reduce mortality. If secondary diseases become a problem, antibiotic therapy may be required, but this should be kept to a minimum.

After marketing a diseased flock, the farm should be completely depopulated of all species of birds. All litter and unused feed must be discarded and the building and equipment thoroughly cleaned and disinfected. Fumigation with formaldehyde is recommended if possible. (This is a hazardous procedure and must not be administered by inexperienced personnel.)

The building should be left vacant for 3 weeks. Vaccines are available in some countries, although they have not been introduced into Canada. Control of rodents, insects and wild birds is also important in the control of infectious disease.

Use of Livestock Medicines on the Dairy Farm

The use of livestock medicines on the dairy farm by producers and veterinarians is important for disease prevention and control.

Management practices which prevent disease will reduce the need for drug treatment. Planned animal health and production programs commit the milk producer, the veterinarian and other herd advisors to the implementation of herd management policies which optimize health and production. However, when needed, medicines must be used responsibly.

This Factsheet provides recommendations on dairy cattle treatment, product label interpretation, treatment recording and antibiotic residue testing of milk. Information about the storage and handling of livestock medicines can be found in the Factsheet "Storage and Handling of Livestock Medicines on the Dairy Farm", Agdex 410/ 662.

Labelling

It is essential to read and understand drug labels to use medications safely and effectively. All livestock medicines bear labels which describe product information, indications for use, dosage, route of administration, warnings and storage instructions.

Product information includes:

- the product name ("brand name"),
- the name of the manufacturer or distributor,
- the drug identification number (D.I.N.),
- the manufacturers lot number,
- the active ingredient in the product, and
- the concentration of active ingredient.

Information provided by the label on product usage includes:

- the indications for medicine use, such as:
- the species (cattle, horses, swine)
- the class of livestock (lactating cows, nonlactating cows, calves) and,
- the disease conditions (mastitis, foot rot, metritis),
- the directions for medicine use, such as
- the dosage (how much, how often and for how long), and,
- the method of administration

  - o intramuscular-into the muscle,
  - o subcutaneous-under the skin,
  - o oral-by mouth,
  - o intramammary-into the udder through the teat end,
  - o intrauterine-into the uterus,
- storage requirements such as refrigeration, and
- the expiry date, the date past which the product should not be used.

All licensed products carry labels with warnings, cautions or precautions about the use of the product. For example, when an antibiotic product is recommended for use in cattle the label may include a warning statement "Warning: Not for use in lactating animals". This means that the product is for use only in non-lactating cattle such as dry cows and heifers. Products licensed for use in lactating cattle will indicate a with-holding time for milk following the last treatment. Products recommended for use in cattle will have a pre-slaughter withholding time on the label. With-holding times for milk and meat will only be valid if the product is used according to label instructions.

Labels may also provide information about disease management or product safety under the "Caution(s)" section. For example, a product recommended for intramuscular administration under directions for usage, may carry a caution that it is "not to be given intravenously" if the product is not safely given by that route. For further interpretation of the cautions, precautions or warnings on a product label consult your veterinarian.

Inserts included with many products provide additional information such as side effects which may occur following product use in some animals. The inserts may contain scientific and medical terms which require interpretation by a veterinarian. Carefully read and understand all insert information before using the product.

Veterinarians must meet the same labelling requirements when drugs are dispensed in non-original containers. Information must be provided which identifies the product, the species and class of animals on which the product is to be used, directions for use and with-holding times. As well, the label must carry the name of the veterinary clinic and the veterinarian prescribing the product.

Drug labels are only useful to those who read them. Make a habit of reading the label before every use of a livestock medicine.

Extra-label Drug Use

"Extra-label" drug use is the use of a drug in any manner other than that listed on the label. Examples of extra-label use include:

- using a product to treat a lactating cow when the label does not list lactating dairy cattle
- using a product at a higher dosage than that listed on the label,
- using a product labelled for intramuscular injection as a subcutaneous injection, and
- using a drug to treat mastitis when the label recommends it only for use in the treatment of respiratory disease.

Extra-label drug use is permitted only under the supervision of a veterinarian. The with-holding time given on the medicine label does not apply when a drug is used in an extra-label manner. The veterinarian advising extra-label use of a livestock medicine is responsible for recommending a proper with-holding time for milk and meat.

Chapter 6

Drug Treatment

Livestock medicines are an important tool in the treatment and prevention of disease. Correct treatment methods assure the safety of food products and insure an effective response to treatment.

Consider the following points before treating dairy cattle.

Selection of Cases

Drug treatment is not always the best option for controlling animal disease. Treat animals based on the diagnosis, the expected response to treatment and the economic benefit expected. For example, viral infections do not respond to antibiotic therapy while those caused by bacteria will. Treating subclinical mastitis at dry off is effective and economical while treating cows during lactation may not be. Select suitable cases to treat with the help and advice of the veterinary practitioner.

Drug Selection

Select the correct therapy. Consult your veterinarian for advice on the correct medication, the route of treatment, the treatment dosage, the time between treatments and the number of treatments. Veterinarians should leave clear written instructions with the herd owner identifying the treated animal and giving information on the treatment protocol. The veterinarian also plays an important role in monitoring the response to treatment.

Treatment Method

Treatment must be given correctly to be effective and to prevent complications. Use the following guidelines to develop good treatment habits.

- Wash your hands before and after handling livestock medicines.
- Use proper equipment: Choose the correct syringe and needle size for the dosage and the type of injection to be given.

For intramuscular injection use a I 1/2", 16 or 18 gauge needle to insure the drug goes in the muscle and not under the skin. Before injecting, pull back on the plunger to insure the needle tip is not in a blood vessel. Select appropriate injection sites with the help of your veterinarian. Read the label for the maximum amount to be injected in one site.

For subcutaneous injection use a 1/2" to 1", 16 or 18 gauge needle. Check that the needle tip is moveable. Inject a small amount of drug to see if a "bleb" of skin starts to rise in the area of the needle tip. This will verify that the needle is under the skin and not in the muscle. Inject only in sites recommended by your veterinarian.

- inject only in clean body sites.
- Use clean equipment. Single use, sterile, disposable needles and syringes are preferred.
- Give repeated injections in different body sites.
- Before infusing antibiotics into the udder, wash and dry your hands and the teat with single use paper towels. Disinfect the teat end with the alcohol swab provided in the medication package. Avoid touching the infusion canula at the end of the treatment tube. Use only single dose infusion products in disposable syringes. Teat dip the teat after infusion of medication.

Dosage Calculation

To calculate the correct dosage you must know the weight of the animal and the dosage rate. For example, to treat a 600 kg cow with procaine penicillin at the label dosage of 2.5 mL per 100 kg of body weight once daily, inject: 600 kg/100 x 2.5 mL = 15 mL.

One milliliter (ml) and one cubic centimetre (cc) represent the same volume and are interchangeable in calculating drug dosages.

Repeat Treatments

Determine the number of treatments to be given from the product label or as recommended by the veterinarian. The duration of treatment should result in a cure without risk of relapse, yet be short enough to insure withholding times are not extended.

Withholding Times

Withholding times for milk and meat are given on product labels. A withdrawal day is a full 24 hours starting after the time of treatment. A 48 hour withdrawal time for milk is illustrated.

Errors in calculating withdrawal times of only a few hours could result in a residue violation. Label withdrawals are not accurate if products are used in an extra-label fashion, if drugs are used in combination (for example intramammary and intramuscular treatments for mastitis given at the same time), or if the treated animal is severely sick and unable to clear the drug from its body at normal rates.

In these cases you must test the milk before addition to the bulk tank to insure it is residue free.

Prevent Residues

Simple management practices will prevent contamination of milk or meat. To prevent residues:

- record all treatments given;
- mark all treated cows;
- inform all people involved in milking of treated cows;
- milk treated cows last or use separate “bypass” equipment to insure that no contaminated milk enters the milk supply;
- discard milk from all quarters of treated cows;
- discard milk from all cows calving within 30 or 42 days of dry treatment according to label directions;
- discard milk from fresh cows for the required period if dry treatment was used;
- use antibiotic test kits as needed;
- and follow label directions for all medications used. These include feed additives, medicated feeds such as calf starter, topical preparations, as well as injectable and infusion products.

Treatment Records

Many antibiotic residue violations result from failure to: identify treated cows, maintain treatment records, and use proper milk withholding times. The record system must make all staff involved in milking aware of treated cows and the period for withholding milk from sale. Identify treated cows in a manner clearly visible to the person milking. Some methods used are:

- leg bands,
- coloured tape or fluorescent hockey tape around the legs or tail, or
- paint markings on the cow’s flank, rump or legs.

In larger herds identification may be colour coded to show the last day to withhold milk. In tie-stall barns where cows always occupy the same stall, coloured tape or tags attached to the milk inlet of the pipeline can identify a treated animal. Reinforce cow identification systems with a prominent chalk board or bulletin board in the milking parlour or barn entrance. Walls constructed of "white board" designed to be written on with special markers are an excellent way to create a very large bulletin board. The identity of all treated cows and the date and time of the last milking withheld should be clearly visible. Train all staff involved in milking to refer to this board immediately before each milking.

Keep a permanent, detailed treatment record for reference and management purposes. Write this in the herd health book or in the individual cow record files. This record should identify the animal, the product and dosage administered, the date of treatment and the milk withholding period. Before shipping any animal for slaughter, check this record to insure pre-slaughter treatment withholding requirements are met.

In addition, store product inserts and packaging from all livestock medicines in a file folder. This "box top file" will provide additional information if questions about previous treatments arise.

On-Farm Antibiotic Testing

The persistence of antibiotic residue in milk of treated cows may vary. This may depend on the cow, her metabolism, the medicine type, the use of a combination of medications, the dosage of medication and the method of administration. Test milk suspected of contamination using antibiotic test kits. Examples of these situations where milk contamination may occur include:

- the addition of purchased milking cows to the herd for which the treatment history is unknown,
- fresh cows purchased during their dry period who have unknown dry off dates or dry treatment histories, cows treated in an extra-label manner, cows treated with more than one product, cows which are severely ill at the time of treatment,
- cows which calve before the end of the milk withholding time following dry treatment,
- establishing the identity of a treated cow when an error in identification may have occurred, and

- the testing of milk in the bulk tank when contamination with milk containing medication may have occurred.

A variety of kits are commercially available. When selecting a test kit the user should recognise that kits vary in the type of antibiotics and amount of antibiotic they detect. No single kit can detect all commonly used antibiotics. Before selecting a test kit confirm with your Ontario Ministry of Agriculture and Food,

Dairy Inspection Branch field person that the kit is comparable in sensitivity to official tests. For the penicillin group of antibiotics the "Delvotest P" is easy to read and detects these drugs at levels similar to the official test.

Milk producers who are comfortable using these tests are encouraged to purchase a test kit for on-farm use. Antibiotic testing services may also be available from veterinarians, milk processing plants, and others. Local staff of the Dairy Inspection Branch have current information on test kits and are also available to conduct a field test on request.

Disposing of Milk From Treated Cows

All unmarketable milk must be disposed of in a manner which protects the environment and keeps drug residues out of all food products. Milk from treated cows can be fed to replacement dairy calves older than 6 weeks of age without harm. Do not feed variable or abnormally large amounts of milk to calves to dispose of it. Milk from treated cows cannot be used in a sour colostrum program since antibiotics prevent normal fermentation. Do not feed milk from treated cows to bull calves or other livestock which may be sold or slaughtered before they are residue free.

Milk from treated cows can be added to a liquid manure storage, or along with straw to absorb it, to a solid manure storage. Do not add milk containing antibiotic to milk house wash water entering a septic tank or treatment trench system. Milk solids will plug the trench tile.

Summary

The ultimate responsibility for insuring a milk supply free of drug residues lies with the milk producer. Use of livestock medicines is a privilege which livestock owners cannot afford to abuse. Correct usage of livestock medicines, recording of treatments, and clearly identifying treated cows are essential practices.

Review the use of livestock medicines on your farm. Use the recommendations of this factsheet to revise procedures to insure the safety and well-being of livestock, the dairy industry and of consumers of dairy products.

Nitrate Poisoning in Cattle, Sheep and Goats

Nitrate poisoning is a condition which may affect ruminants consuming certain forages or water that contain an excessive amount of nitrate.

Causes of Nitrate Poisoning

Under normal conditions, nitrate ingested by ruminant livestock, like cattle, sheep and goats, is converted to ammonia and then bacterial protein in the rumen by bacteria. The steps of conversion in this process are as follows:

—BactProtein—Nitrate (NO_3) → Nitrite (NO_2) → Ammonia (NH_3) → Amino Acid → Protein

Nitrate is converted to nitrite faster than nitrite is converted to ammonia. Consequently, when higher than normal amounts of nitrate are consumed, an accumulation of nitrite may occur in the rumen. Nitrite then will be absorbed into the bloodstream and will convert hemoglobin to methemoglobin, which is unable to transport oxygen. Thus, when an animal dies from nitrate poisoning, it is due to a lack of oxygen.

The occurrence of nitrate poisoning is difficult to predict because nitrate levels can change rapidly in plants and the toxicity of nitrate varies greatly among livestock due to age, health status, and diets. However, concern should certainly be raised when plant growth has been less than half of normal or nitrogen application more than twice recommended.

Nitrate Levels in Plants

Plants normally take up nitrogen from the soil in the form of nitrate, regardless of the form of nitrogen fertilizer (including manure) applied. However little nitrate accumulates in plants, when growth is normal, because the plant stem and leaves rapidly convert nitrate to plant amino acids and protein. Under certain conditions, however, this balance can be disrupted so that the roots will take up nitrate faster than the plant can convert the nitrate to protein.

The nitrate-to-protein cycle in a plant is dependent on three factors:

- Adequate water
- Energy from sunlight
- A temperature conducive to rapid chemical reactions.

If any one of these factors is inadequate, the root continues to absorb nitrate at the same rate while storing it unchanged in the stalk and lower parts of the leaves. When this situation develops, nitrate accumulates.

Nitrates may also accumulate in plants from excessive nitrogen fertilization, for example on fields where a large amount of manure have been applied.

Some plants are more likely to accumulate nitrate that others. Crops capable of high levels of nitrate accumulation under adverse conditions include corn, small grains, sudangrass, and sorghum. Weeds capable of nitrate accumulation include pigweed, lambs quarter, sunflower, bindweed and many others. Vegetables capable of accumulating large amounts of nitrate that are most frequently grazed include sugar beets, lettuce, cabbage, potatoes and carrots.

Nitrates in Water

Nitrates and nitrites are water soluble. They move with the water. Any nitrate added to, or produced within, the soil may be leached or washed away by moving water—either by surface run-off or ground water percolation.

Nitrates are more concentrated below or near the area of waste accumulation or disposal such as manure piles, feedlots, septic tank disposal fields, cesspools, privies, etc. Excess nitrates also are more apt to be found in ground water under low areas and waterways that collect or convey

Water samples from shallow, dug, bored and driven wells more frequently contain excess nitrates than water from deeper, drilled wells. Nitrate levels generally are highest following wet periods and lowest, even down to zero nitrates, during dry periods which may cause a false sense of security. Preferably, a well should be tested immediately following a wet period.

Toxicity Variation

Ruminant livestock can tolerate a wide range of nitrate, depending on several factors. Factors making nitrate less toxic include:

- The animal can become conditioned to eat larger amounts of feed with high nitrate content if the increase is gradual.

- Healthy animals are less likely to be adversely affected than animals in poor health.
- Adequate amounts of available carbohydrates (grain) allow the animal to consume more nitrate because carbohydrates enhance the conversion process from nitrate to microbial protein.

Factors making nitrate more toxic include:

- Rapid diet changes can trigger nitrate poisoning.
- Parasitism or other conditions causing anemia will increase susceptibility.
- Nitrate in more than one diet component (e.g. water and forage).

Symptoms of Nitrate Problems

Many general symptoms such as poor appetite, weak calves, lambs or kids, abortions, poor growth, and general unthrifty conditions are frequently blamed on nitrate. These and other general problems can also be caused by a number of disease, nutritional or managerial problems. Therefore, it is essential to study the situation thoroughly before concluding that nitrate is the problem.

Simple chronic nitrate toxicity is rare. More likely, high nitrate is only one of several factors resulting in poor performance. For example, poor performance on a ration that is low in energy or lacking in essential minerals is apt to be worse if nitrate is also present. When good feeding and management practices are followed, it is very difficult to produce chronic nitrate problems.

Many factors have been suggested to explain the different results obtained in research trials studying the nitrate problem. Age, condition, and species of the animal, other chemical compounds and nutrients in the ration, and the types of nitrogen compounds in the feed or water are some of the factors that must be considered.

The most dramatic nitrate toxicity problems have occurred when hungry cattle were put on corn stalks, oat straw or weedy pasture. Under these conditions the highest nitrate feeds are fed as the total ration, and the feeding of well-balanced rations and adaptation by the animal are ignored. Sudden change to high nitrate corn silage as the main feed can cause problems. Milking cows and other animals receiving large amounts of grain are not as likely to have nitrate toxicity problems as dry cows, heifers and other animals because the milking cows are on a higher energy ration and because the high nitrate feedstuff is likely to be a smaller proportion of the total diet..

Grains and other concentrates are low in nitrate. Forages (leaves and stems) will accumulate more nitrate than grains. Because forage comprises a larger percentage of ruminants dies, high nitrate in feed is more likely to be of concern in feeding ruminants than non-ruminants. However, nitrate from feed or water can cause problems for all animals and to humans.

Taking an Accurate Sample for Analysis

If fresh-chopped forage or silage is suspected of being high in nitrates, it should be tested. Samples can be analysed by some commercial forage testing laboratories as well as by the University of Wisconsin Soil & Forage Analysis Lab (8396 Yellowstone Dr., Marshfield, WI, 54449) and the Soil & Plant Analysis Lab (8452 Mineral Point Rd., Verona, WI, 53593).

The two key steps to getting accurate nitrate analysis are:

1. To make sure the sample is representative of the feed or water that is being analysed.
2. To prevent loss of the nitrate between sampling and laboratory analysis.

Preventing Nitrate Loss in the Sample

Preventing nitrate loss in the sample before analysis is critical to getting accurate results. This is difficult in silages and fresh forages therefore it is best to take fresh silages and samples directly to the laboratory. If samples must be held or shipped, samples should be frozen or dried before shipment. Freeze samples in airtight, plastic bags for at least 24 hours and ship in insulated containers to reach the laboratory while still frozen. (DO NOT ship samples late in the week to risk getting delayed over the weekend.)

Alternatively, dry samples by spreading in a thin layer on clean paper to dry. Artificial heat is desirable, but the sample should not get above 160° F. Fresh forages will ferment in airtight bags and for this reason are usually dried. Silage samples are usually frozen because it is difficult to dry without losing volatile materials.

Water samples should be collected in special water sample bottles obtained from the laboratory or from the health agency in the area. To obtain a good sample of water from a well, let the water run until water in pipes and pressure tank has been discharged. It is comparatively easy to get a good water sample and the laboratory analysis is also more standardised. There is less variation in test results from water than feed. However, nitrate levels in water can vary considerably from month to month.

Results of analysis on the same sample of feed can vary considerably due to limitations of chemical test used. Variations of 100 parts per million in a feed are well within the range of expected errors. Results of tests on feeds containing small amounts of nitrate might appear large but could be within the normal tolerance of test used. For example, if a report on one sample of silage shows 200 parts per million of NO_3-N and another report shows 300 ppm of NO_3-N, they are for all practical purposes the same. If reported as percent, the variation does not appear as large. In the above example, the percent NO_3-N is.02 and.03.

Interpreting and Using Nitrate Reports

Results of nitrate analysis may be confusing because of the variation in methods of reporting. In the chemical analysis for nitrate, the actual element determined is the oxidised nitrogen. However, values may be reported as percent nitrate (NO_3), or nitrate-nitrogen (NO_3-N). Efforts have been made to have nitrate analysis and tolerances for safety uniformly reported as nitrate-nitrogen on 100 percent dry matter basis. However, at present, reports may be given as nitrate or nitrate-nitrogen and may be reported as either percent or as parts per million (ppm).

Toxic Effects of Nitrate

With all the biological variation that can exist in both plants and animals, it is obviously difficult to develop specific guidelines that fit all conditions. Safe levels of nitrate are not specifically known for all the various livestock feeding conditions. At the same time, some general guidelines are needed. The concept in developing the tables that follow is to be conservative to help assure safety. At the same time, reasonable feeding and care of the animal is assumed. There are two kinds of possible toxicity that are of concern: (1) Acute or lethal and (2) Chronic or non-lethal.

Uggestions for Minimising Nitrate Problems

Toxicity or safety of a feed containing more than normal amounts of nitrate involves many factors. These include total daily intake of nitrate, previous adaptation of the animal to high nitrate, feeding practices, nutritional quality of the ration and general health of the animal. In addition, the nitrate level of the water may be a contributing factor.

The following are the major factors that influence possible nitrate problems. Preventing or changing a condition that increases the problem will help decrease or prevent the problem.

Total nitrate intake is the critical problem rather than the amount in any one feed in the ration. For example, a dangerous level in a feed that makes up the total ration could be perfectly safe if it comprised only half the ration. Likewise, a safe level in the feed may be a problem if the water also contains high levels of nitrate.

Determine nitrate in all suspicious feeds and in the water. Limit the amount of any questionable feed. Forages, especially corn and oat silages, green chop or pasture and weeds, are the most common sources of the problem. Limits may need to be greater if the water also contains significant nitrate levels.

Nitrate in one dose may be very toxic while the same amount divided into several smaller doses is perfectly safe. For example, in one study, giving a 1000 pound cow 150 grams (about 5 ounces) of nitrate (NO_3) in one dose produced acute toxicity. Spraying three times as much, or 450 grams (about one pound) of nitrate on the hay consumed in a day, did not produce acute toxicity.

If a feed contains questionable amounts of nitrate, divide the daily feeding into smaller feedings. For example, feed ten pounds of silage 3 or 4 times per day rather than feeding 30 or 40 pounds at one feeding.

Nitrate is not normally accumulated in the animal because it is continually converted to other nitrogen compounds that are utilised or excreted in the urine and feces. The ability to utilise and effectively excrete the nitrogen compounds requires adaptation by the animal. A toxic level given to a cow that had been on a very low nitrate intake could be a safe level if the same amount had been gradually added to the ration. If a toxic level is fed repeatedly, liver and kidney damage can occur.

If a feed is questionable, feed a small amount for a week; if no problem is noted the amount can be increased. When changing to a new feed or different source of feed, it is always better to make the change gradually.

Safe utilisation of nitrate requires general good nutrition and proper rumen function in cattle, sheep and goats. Rumen micro-organisms require readily available carbohydrate, protein and minerals. Additional vitamin A reduces the toxic effects of nitrates in poultry.

Feed a balanced ration. Liberal feeding of a good grain mix insures adequate levels of energy and protein. Minerals should be provided in the grain mixture, as well as by free choice feeding of trace mineral salt and a calcium-phosphorus supplement. Nitrates might destroy or interfere with the conversion of carotene to vitamin A; therefore, the use of a protein source that contains vitamin A or adding a vitamin A supplement in some way is generally advised when high nitrate feeds are used. Avoid feeding high nitrate feeds to animals that are unthrifty or sick for any reason. Do not feed questionable forages to cows that have impaired rumen function. Elimination of high nitrate feeds from rations for dry and recently early lactation cows is also a good practice.

Nitrates can accumulate in plants when adverse growing conditions such as drought, hot weather, cool weather or frost slows the growth of the plants. Cool season crops such as small grains and permanent forage grasses may accumulate nitrates in hot, dry weather while warm season crops such as corn and sorghums can accumulate nitrates when the temperatures are low or when growth has been arrested due to frost.

Nitrates primarily accumulate in the lower stems and leaves of corn, sorghums, small grains, grasses and weeds. They seldom accumulate at sufficiently high concentrations to be a problem in legumes. If the nitrates are suspected to be a problem, avoid harvesting the basal portions of the plant. Avoid pasturing hungry animals or green feeding on drought stunted crops or weedy pastures. Place suspect crops in the silo and allow to ferment for one to three months before feeding and then follow suggestions given previously. Ensiling will allow conversion of nitrate to ammonia and may reduce nitrate levels by 30 to 50%. Haymaking does not reduce the nitrate level of the forage.

Nitrates are hazardous to man. Silo gases are a common cause of both chronic and acute respiratory problems to farmers. When plants are high in nitrate at time of ensiling, various nitrogen gases are formed. Nitrogen dioxide is a brownish yellow gas with a bleach-like odour, that is sometimes seen coming down the silo chute or is layered on top of the silo below closed doors. The gas is heavier than air so it accumulates in low enclosed areas. Nitrogen dioxide is potentially very dangerous to man and animals.

Don't leave the silo room door open to the barn as the gas may come down from the silo and kill animals in the barn overnight. Be sure to ventilate a recently filled silo before entering it by running the blower for several minutes. Open outside doors or windows near bottom of the silo chute and use fan to force gas outside. Escaping nitrogen in the form of gas from the silo reduces nitrate content of silage. Presence of the yellow gas during filling does not mean the silage will be dangerous as a feed, however, it is good evidence that high nitrate was present. Therefore, this silage should be checked for nitrate before feeding.

Highly Pathogenic H5N1 Avian Influenza and Pets

Can Highly Pathogenic H5N1 Infect Pets?

The highly pathogenic Asian Strain of H5N1 avian influenza (AI) currently found in Asia, Africa and Europe can infect multiple species of domestic (chickens, turkeys, quails, guinea fowl, etc.) wild and pet birds. This virus has also been detected in mammalian species including humans, rats and mice, weasels and ferrets, pigs, cats and dogs.

However, the number of documented cases of AI H5N1 in non-avian species is very low despite the fact that this virus has caused large avian outbreaks globally, over the last few years.

How is it Transmitted?

It is believed that the vast majority of human cases of H5N1 Asian strain of AI are the result of direct and close contact with infected birds. There have been no documented or reported cases of AI H5N1 being transmitted to humans from mammalian pets.

To date, the only feral cats shown conclusively to be naturally infected with AI H5N1 were found in an area of Germany which experienced a significant outbreak in wild birds in February, 2006. It is suspected that these cats became infected after eating infected wild birds.

There have been additional reports of increased mortality in cats during AI H5N1 outbreaks in other countries but these have not been substantiated by laboratory tests. Some non-domestic cats (tigers and leopards) have also contracted the disease in zoos after eating raw infected poultry meat.

Serological studies in several Asian countries suggest that dogs have been exposed to the virus. An unpublished study carried out in 2005 by the National Institute of Animal Health in Bangkok showed that 160 out of 629 village dogs (25%) had antibodies to AI H5N1. No clinical cases of AI H5N1 have been reported in dogs.

Can Infected Animals, Such as Cats, Transmit the Virus to Humans?

The World Organisation for Animal Health and the Food and Agriculture Organisation of the United Nations confirm the statement issued by the World Health Organisation (WHO) in February 2006 that "there is no present evidence that domestic cats can play a role in the transmission cycle of H5N1 viruses".

Current science suggests that the risk of a human being contracting AI from a mammalian pet is very low. Nonetheless, owners are encouraged to take appropriate precautions to protect their pets and themselves. Pet owners should contact their veterinarian if they have any concerns about the health of their pet.

Should Pet Owners Take Special Precautions?

In view of the susceptibility of certain types of cats, it is recommended that cats in infected zones and surveillance zones set up around AI outbreaks be kept indoors. Dogs in these areas should be kept on a leash as a precautionary measure.

Pet birds, if they are not normally kept indoors, should also be restricted to the indoors in areas that are experiencing AI H5N1 outbreaks in domestic or wild birds.

The Food and Agriculture Organisation (FAO) of the United Nations provides the following advice to cat owners in areas where highly pathogenic H5N1 has been diagnosed or suspected in poultry or wild birds:

- be especially vigilant for any dead or sick cats and report such findings to the local veterinarian;
- do not touch or handle any sick looking or dead cat (or other animal) and report to the authorities;
- wash hands with water and soap regularly and especially after handling animals and cleaning their litter boxes or coming in contact with feces or saliva;
- make sure contact between cats and wild birds or poultry (or the feces) is avoided, and/or keep cats inside;
- if cats bring a sick or dead bird inside the house, put on plastic gloves and dispense of the bird in plastic bags for collection by local veterinary animal handlers;
- keep stray cats outside the house and avoid contact with them; and

- if cats show breathing problems or nasal discharge, a veterinarian should be consulted.

It must be stressed that pets should not be abandoned under any circumstances. In some countries there has been public fear and uncertainty about the health of pets, mostly cats, and their role in spreading AI H5N1. Pets have been given up and abandoned as a result of these concerns. This seriously compromises the welfare of the animal through starvation and exposure to accidental injury and disease.

Bordetella Bronchiseptica

Bordetella bronchiseptica is a small, gram-negative, rod-shaped bacterium of the genus *Bordetella.* It can cause infectious bronchitis, but rarely infects humans. Closely related to *B. pertussis*—the obligate human pathogen that causes pertussis or *whooping cough—B. bronchiseptica* can persist in the environment for extended periods.

Pathogenesis

Humans are not natural carriers of B. bronchiseptica, which typically infects the respiratory tracts of smaller mammals (cats, dogs, rabbits, etc). People are more likely to be infected by B. pertussis or B. parapertussis.

B. bronchiseptica does not express pertussis toxin, which is one of the characteristic virulence factors of B. pertussis. But it has the genes to do so, highlighting the close evolutionary relationship between the two species.

Veterinary Pathogenesis

In veterinary medicine, *B. bronchiseptica* leads to a range of pathologies in different hosts. It is a serious disease of dogs, pigs, and rabbits and has been seen in cats, horses, and seals. There is a PCR test for the pathogen.

In pigs, *B. bronchiseptica* and *Pasteurella multocida* act synergistically to cause atrophic rhinitis, a disease resulting in arrested growth and distortion of the turbinates in the nasal terminus (snout).

In dogs, *B. bronchiseptica* causes acute tracheobronchitis, which typically has a harsh, honking cough. Kennel cough can also be caused by canine adenovirus-2 or canine parainfluenza virus or a combination of pathogens.

In rabbits, *B. bronchiseptica* is often found in the nasal tract. It is often assumed to cause a nearly asymptomatic infection known as snuffles, but the causative agent for that disease is *Pasteurella multocida*; "*B. bronchiseptica*" often co-infects the nasal passage at the same time.

Bronchiseptica

Cats infected with *B. bronchiseptica* have been seen with tracheobronchitis, conjunctivitis and rhinitis (upper-respiratory tract infection or URI), mandibular lymphadenopathy, and pneumonia. However, URI in cats can also be caused by herpesvirus, calicivirus, *Mycoplasma* species, or *Chlamydia psittaci*. An intranasal vaccine exists for cats.

Prevention and Control of Bordetella Bronchiseptica Infection in Cats

Until now prevention of feline upper respiratory tract disease (URTD) has been limited to cattery management.

Particularly good hygiene practices and the reduction of stress in cats, is an important aid in the prevention of URTD in cats. Removal of chronically-infected cats from affected catteries can also be considered.

An intranasal vaccine is now available in some countries and this can be used to help prevent URTD outbreaks in catteries. Vaccination is also indicated to help prevent respiratory disease in cats which:

- come into contact with other cats and dogs
- are boarded at catteries or are exhibited.

Cat vaccination programmes should always be combined with good husbandry: good nutrition, sanitation, ventilation, parasite control and control of other respiratory pathogens to minimise the occurrence of clinical disease. During parturition, queens may pass *Bordetella bronchiseptica* to their offspring; kittens obtained from breeding catteries and rescue shelters are, therefore, particularly at risk from this disease. Since *Bordetella bronchiseptica* infection in kittens can cause acute death as a result of bronchopneumonia, this risk must be taken seriously. The potential for mortality and the general morbidity caused by infectious URTD warrants the use of measures designed to tackle disease, particularly in high-risk animals. Intranasal Vaination is an important part of such preventative schemes.

Good Cattery Practice and Prevention

Bordetella bronchiseptica (Bb) infection can be prevented by a combination of good cattery practice, careful management and vaccination. *Bb* does not survive long outside the cat and is killed by many common disinfectants so routine hygiene measures are sufficient to prevent disease spreading through the environment.

Recommendations for good cattery practice:

- clean and disinfect cages, food bowls and litter trays on a daily basis e.g. hypochlorite or quaternary ammonium compounds
- use disinfectant baths for foot-dipping in between entering pens
- enter each cage as few times as possible
- finish all cleaning and disinfection tasks in one area before moving on to the next
- disinfect cages thoroughly between cats, preferably leaving empty for 2 days
- put cats with any previous respiratory problems or suspected carrier cats at one end of the cattery and feed last
- avoid overcrowding: provide one pen per cat wherever possible (unless the cats come from the same household)
- maintain optimal environmental conditions for comfort: optimum temperature, good ventilation, low relative humidity, good drainage

Infected cats can be treated with antibiotics but blanket treatment of cats in your cattery is needed. This is expensive and carrier cats may still shed *Bb* and infect healthy cats. This form of control can encourage the development of antibiotic resistance. Good cattery practice requires veterinary advice on vaccination programmes aimed to prevent feline URTD.

Streptococcal Infection in Poultry

Species are the cause of opportunistic infections in poultry leading to acute and chronic conditions in affected birds. Disease varies according to the Streptococcal species but common presentations include septicaemia, peritonitis, salpingitis and endocarditis.

Common species affecting poultry include:

- *S. gallinaceus* in broiler chickens
- *S. gallolyticus* which is a pathogen of racing pigeons and turkey poults
- *S. dysgalactiae* in broiler chickens

- *S. mutans* in geese
- *S. pluranimalium* in broiler chickens
- *S. equi subsp. zooepidemicus* in chickens and turkeys
- *S. suis* in psittacine birds.

Diagnosis

Post-mortem findings include friable internal organs, abdominal effusion and evidence of sepsis in the joints, heart valves and brain.

Bacteria can usually be cultured from tissues collected at necropsy or identified by microscope examination.

Treatment and Control

The organism should be cultured and antibiotic sensitivity should be determined before treatment is started. Amoxycillin is usually effective in treating streptococcal infections.

Biosecurity protocols and good hygiene are important in preventing the disease.

Vaccination is available against S. gallolyticus *and can also protect pigeons.*

Streptococcus & Enterococcus Infections-Poultry

Introduction

Streptococcal and enterococcal infections in poultry can cause acute septicaemia and chronic infections in affected birds.

There are ~50 recognised members of the Streptococcus genus and 21 of Enterococcus spp. all are commensal organisms, primarily of the gastrointestinal tract and mucosal surfaces, in both animals and humans. Some are also ubiquitous in the environment.

The majority of infections from these pathogens are opportunistic.

There does not appear to be any zoonotic risk to humans from ingestion of infected birds with these infections, with the exception of Streptococcus suis which is rare in birds and more commonly acquired from pigs. There are however concerns regarding the spread of Vancomycin Resistant Enterococci (VRE) to humans from poultry.

Diseases—Streptococcosis

Thus clinical signs also vary widely and may range from anorexia, lethargy and diarrhoea to high mortality rates and severe neurological signs, lameness or jaundice.

Many other species not discussed here have been isolated from healthy birds and are thought to be non-pathogenic.

Known as a facultative pathogen in racing pigeons causing acute mortality, lameness, weight loss, diarrhoea and inability to fly. Also causes mortality in turkey poults.

Associated with endocarditis, peritonitis, salpingitis, egg drop, septicaemia and high mortality in chickens and also massive mortality in eared grebes. In turkeys, the same pathogen is thought to be responsible for septicaemia.

Enterococcosis

Enterococci are frequently involved in infections of day old chicks, affecting primarily the yolk sac.

Lesions

On necropsy, changes in chickens, ducks and turkeys are similar and various organs may be affected, dependent of the species involved. Septicaemic birds are the most common presentation, in which the liver is pale and friable and viscera within both abdominal and thoracic cavities are congested with yellow or orange-ish discolouration. There may be a sero-fibrinous or serosanguinous exudate covering some organs. The skin may be discoloured and crusting in cases of cellulitis/ dermatitis and joint lesions possibly with yellow caseous exudates occur in septic arthritis. Vegetative lesions are indicative of endocarditis. Infarcts can be present in any organ. In birds with encephalomalacia, lesions may be found anywhere except the cerebellum and yellow discolourations will be seen; malacia and heterophilic infiltration are visible microscopically. Pectoral muscle necrosis is pathognomic for S. gallolyticus septicaemia in pigeons.

Diagnosis

Isolation and identification is essential for confirmed diagnosis. Bacteriology can be performed on yolk, embryo fluid, valvular vegetations from necropsy, blood samples from septicaemic birds, joint and any suspected lesions. It is thought that capillary microblood cultures may be more sensitive due to trapping of the micro-organisms in these small vessels.

The pathogens can then be cultured on sheep or ox blood agar, selective blood agar or MacConkey agar. Serological Lancefield testing can also be performed on beta haemolytic colonies.

The organism can often be visualised in microscopic sections as generic gram positive cocci.

Treatment

Culture and sensitivity should always be performed whenever possible before selecting treatment. The efficacy of treatment deteriorates with progression of disease within a flock. Chronic cases, especially those involving endocarditis and arthritis, often do not respond.

Amoxycillin appears to be the drug of first choice for most infections according to sensitivity studies in poultry.

Ampicillin, doxycycline and erythromycin are effective in pigeon outbreaks of S. gallolyticus.

Control

Good hygiene, management and housing strategies are imperative. Hygiene in the hatcher is particularly important to prevent iatrogenic transmission. It is possible to transmit these opportunistic bacteria when giving vaccinations, e.g. those for Mareks Disease. Minimisation of stress and immunosuppressive disease is also key.

Vaccines are available against S. gallolyticus *and provide a degree of clinical protection for pigeons.*

Manual of Diagnostic Tests and Vaccines for Terrestrial Animals

The *Manual of Diagnostic Tests and Vaccines for Terrestrial Animals* (*Terrestrial Manual*) aims to facilitate international trade in animals and animal products and to contribute to the improvement of animal health services world-wide. The principal target readership is laboratories carrying out veterinary diagnostic tests and surveillance, plus vaccine manufacturers and regulatory authorities in Member Countries. The objective is to provide internationally agreed diagnostic laboratory methods and requirements for the production and control of vaccines and other biological products.

This ambitious task has required the cooperation of highly renowned animal health specialists from many countries. The OIE, the World Organisation for Animal Health, is clearly the most appropriate organisation to undertake this task on a global level. The main activities of the organisation, which was established in 1924 and in 2008 comprised 172 Member Countries and Territories, are as follows:

1. To ensure transparency in the global animal disease and zoonosis situation.

2. To collect, analyse and disseminate scientific veterinary information on animal disease control methods.
3. To provide expertise and encourage international solidarity in the control of animal diseases.
4. Within its mandate under the WTO (World Trade Organisation) Agreement on Sanitary and Phytosanitary Measures (SPS Agreement), to safeguard world trade by publishing health standards for international trade in animals and animal products.
5. To improve the legal framework and resources of national Veterinary Services.
6. To provide a better guarantee of the safety of food of animal origin and to promote animal welfare through a science-based approach.

The *Terrestrial Manual*, covering infectious and parasitic diseases of mammals, birds and bees, was first published in 1989. Each successive edition has extended and updated the information provided. This sixth edition includes new chapters on Guidelines for international standards for vaccine banks, Turkey rhinotracheitis (avian metapneumovirus), Small hive beetle infestation (*Aethina tumida*) and camelpox, and *Mycoplasma synoviae* has been added to the chapter on Avian mycoplasmosis (previously the chapter focused on *Mycoplasma gallisepticum*.

As a companion volume to the *Terrestrial Animal Health Code*, the *Terrestrial Manual* sets laboratory standards for all OIE listed diseases as well as several other diseases of global importance. In particular it specifies (in blue font) those "Prescribed Tests" that are recommended for use in health screening for international trade or movement of animals. The *Terrestrial Manual* has become widely adopted as a key reference book for veterinary laboratories around the world. Aquatic animal diseases are included in a separate *Aquatic Manual*.

The task of commissioning chapters and compiling the *Terrestrial Manual* was assigned to the OIE Biological Standards Commission by the International Committee of the OIE (General Assembly of national Delegates of Member Countries and Territories). Manuscripts were requested from specialists in each of the diseases or the other topics covered. After initial scrutiny by the Consultant Technical Editor, the chapters were sent to scientific reviewers and to experts at OIE Reference Laboratories. They were also circulated to all OIE Member Countries for review and comment. The Biological Standards Commission and the Consultant Technical Editor took all the resulting comments into consideration, often referring back to the authors for further help, beforc finalising the chapters. The final text has the approval of the International Committee of the OIE.

A procedure for the official recognition of commercialised diagnostic tests, under the authority of the International Committee, was finalised in September 2004. Data are submitted using a validation template that was developed by the Biological Standards Commission. Submissions are evaluated by appointed experts, who advise the Biological Standards Commission before the final opinion of the OIE International Committee is sought. All information on the submission of applications can be found on the OIE Web site.

Arrangement of the Terrestrial Manual

Terrestrial Manual, contains eleven introductory chapters that deal with a variety of general subjects of interest to veterinary laboratory diagnosticians. These chapters are intended to give a brief introduction to their subjects. They are to be regarded as background information rather than standards.

The main part of the *Terrestrial Manual* (Part 2) covers standards for diagnostic tests and vaccines for the diseases listed in the OIE *Terrestrial Animal Health Code.* The diseases are in alphabetical order, subdivided by animal host species. OIE listed diseases are transmissible diseases that have the potential for very serious and rapid spread, irrespective of national borders. They have particularly serious socio-economic or public health consequences and are of major importance in the international trade of animals and animal products. Four of the diseases in Section 2.9 are included in some individual species sections, but these chapters cover several species and thus give a broader description. Some additional diseases that may also be of importance to trade but that do not have a chapter in the *Terrestrial Code* are also included in Section 2.9. The contributors of all the chapters are listed on pages xxii–xxxv, but the final responsibility for the content of the *Terrestrial Manual* lies with the International Committee of the OIE.

Format of Chapters

Each disease chapter includes a summary intended to provide information for veterinary officials and other readers who need a general overview of the tests and vaccines available for the disease.

This is followed by a text giving greater detail for laboratory workers. In each disease chapter, Part A gives a general introduction to the disease, Part B deals with laboratory diagnosis of the disease, and Part C (where appropriate) with the requirements for vaccines or *in vivo* diagnostic biologicals.

The information concerning production and control of vaccines or diagnostics is given as an example; it is not always necessary to follow these when there are scientifically justifiable reasons for using alternative approaches. Bibliographic references that provide further information are listed at the end of each chapter.

Explanation of the Tests Described and of the Table on Pages xi–xiv

The table on pages xi–xiv lists diagnostic tests in two categories: 'prescribed' and 'alternative'. Prescribed tests are those that are required by the *Terrestrial Animal Health Code* for the testing of animals before they are moved internationally. In the *Terrestrial Manual* these tests are printed in blue. At present it is not possible to have prescribed tests for every listed disease. 'Alternative tests' are those that are suitable for the diagnosis of disease within a local setting, and can also be used in the import/export of animals after bilateral agreement. There are often other tests described in the chapters, which may also be of some practical value in local situations or which may still be under development.

World Animal Health Information

The WAHID Interface provides access to all data held within OIE's new World Animal Health Information System (WAHIS). It replaces and significantly extends the former web interface named Handistatus II System.

A comprehensive range of information is available from:

- Immediate notifications and follow-up reports submitted by Member Countries in response to exceptional disease events occurring in these countries as well as follow-up reports about these events,
- Six-monthly reports describing the OIE-listed disease situations in each country
- Annual reports providing further background information on animal health, on laboratory and vaccine production facilities, etc.

To start, select one of the headings on the left. You can then explore available information

- by country (or group of countries),
- by disease,
- focusing on control measures, or
- comparing the animal health situation between two countries.

Veterinary Medicine

Intute: Veterinary medicine provides free access to high quality resources on the Internet. Each resource has been evaluated and categorised by subject specialists based at UK universities.

No new resources are being added to the catalogue, but existing resources will be checked and broken links will be fixed until July 2011.

Chapter 7

Animal Health Strategy

A Challenging EU Animal Health Strategy

Based on the evaluation results and the stakeholder consultation, the Commission is pleased to present its proposal for a new EU Animal Health Strategy (2007-2013).

This will allow further debate in the EU inter-institutional fora, with Council and the Parliament expected to establish their positions by the end of this year. Overall, the strategy encompasses a challenging 6 year programme of work aimed towards clear outcomes:

- Prioritisation of EU intervention;
- A modern and appropriate animal health framework;
- Better prevention, surveillance and crisis preparedness;
- Science, Innovation and Research.
- The timetable for delivery of all the specific actions included in this strategy will depend on the position of the Council and the Parliament, and also on our human resources capacity.

Vision

Our vision is to work in partnership to increase the prevention of animal health related problems before they happen: "Prevention is better than cure".

Purpose

The strategy provides direction for the development of animal health policy, based on extensive stakeholder consultation and a firm commitment to high standards of animal health. It will facilitate the establishment of priorities that are consistent with agreed strategic goals and the revision of, and agreement on, acceptable and appropriate standards.

Scope of the Strategy

The concept of animal health covers not only the absence of disease in animals, but also the critical relationship between the health of animals and their welfare. It is also a pillar for the Commission's policy on public health and food safety.

The strategy covers the health of all animals in the EU kept for food, farming, sport, companionship, entertainment and in zoos. It also covers wild animals and animals used in research where there is a risk of them transmitting disease to other animals or to humans. The strategy also covers the health of animals transported to, from and within the EU.

The strategy is aimed at the entire EU, including animal owners, the veterinary profession, food chain businesses, animal health industries, animal interest groups, researchers and teachers, governing bodies of sport and recreational organisations, educational facilities, consumers, travellers, competent authorities of Member States and the EU Institutions.

The strategy builds on the current animal health legal framework1 in the EU and the standards and guidelines of the World Organisation for Animal Health (Office international des Epizooties – OIE). It will aim at ensuring consistency with other EU policies and the EU's international commitments.

It will guide the development of new policies or guidelines and will enhance existing animal health arrangements in the Community based on scientific risk assessments and taking into account social, economic and ethical considerations. It will support the achievement of a high level of environmental protection by considering the impacts on the environment in the development of the policy framework.

Goals

The strategy sets out some challenging aims, not just for the EU institutions and Governments, but for all citizens, to improve animal health. The strategy's goals are:Goal 1

- To ensure a high level of public health and food safety by minimising the incidence of biological and chemical risks to humans.Goal
- To promote animal health by preventing/reducing the incidence of animal diseases, and in this way to support farming and the rural economy.Goal

- To improve economic growth/cohesion/competitiveness assuring free circulation of goods and proportionate animal movements.Goal
- To promote farming practices and animal welfare which prevent animal health related threats and minimise environmental impacts in support of the EU Sustainable Development Strategy.

Simple and reliable performance indicators will help to measure progress towards the strategy's goals, guide policy, inform priorities, target resources and focus discussion. They will be developed in consultation with stakeholders and improved over time as better veterinary and other data becomes available. They will cover both hard indicators of animal health (e.g. disease prevalence, number of animals eliminated) and softer indicators tracking the confidence, expectations and perceptions of European citizens. It must be recognised that uncertainties and unforeseeable events may affect achievement of the performance indicators..

The action plan will aim to explain the significant breadth of activity which is being carried out or will be carried out at EU level through legislative proposal or other mechanisms in order to deliver the different strategy goals over the next six years.

The action plan to deliver the strategic goals (section 4) will focus on four main pillars, or areas of activity:

A partnership approach built on trust, openness and a willingness to take difficult decisions is essential for success. The strategy can only bring about real change if everyone involved in animal health works together and with all interested citizens. There are many excellent examples of partnership in action in the current Community Animal Health Policy. We must take advantage of existing collaborations, encourage new initiatives and make more use of non-legislative alternatives to regulation.

An "Animal Health Advisory Committee" will include representatives from non governmental organisations across the animal health sector, consumers and governments. The "Animal Health Advisory Committee" will provide strategic guidance on the appropriate/ acceptable level of animal or public health protection, and on priorities for action and communication. It will also follow the strategy's progress: it will be consulted on all impact assessments and will advise the Commission on the best means of delivering agreed outcomes.

CommUnIC AtIon

Animal health is a concern for all European citizens. This concern stems from the public health and food safety aspects of animal health but also from the economic costs that animal disease outbreaks can trigger and the animal welfare considerations, including the implications of disease control. The Commission is committed to pursue its objectives of clarity and transparency when communicating with consumers and stakeholders what the EU is doing and why. European and national entities need to cooperate to ensure a coherent message and enhance public confidence.

Communicating the Strategy

There will be annual reporting on the strategy's progress and wider communication of policies and initiatives. Communication will take different forms depending on the message that is being delivered and the target audience. It will include participation in international or national events, developing relationships with the media and non governmental organisations.

Communication in Case of Crisis

Good communication on risk to stakeholders/consumers is also of utmost importance, as an incorrect public perception of risk may force the regulator to take unjustified or disproportionate measures in the case of a crisis. The Animal Health Advisory Committee will advise the Commission to further improve communication during a crisis situation.

A new Animal Health Strategy for the European Union (2007-2013) where "Prevention is better than cure"all interested parties in the risk management process to gain the widest possible agreement and shared responsibility for the judgements made and to deliver agreed objectives.

Targets will be set at community level, national level and, where appropriate, regional level. Suitable performance indicators will allow the assessment of progress over the next six years. The appropriate amount of resources to be applied to achieve the desired level of protection, and the development of a responsibility and cost sharing scheme, will be based on the categorisation of biological and chemical risks.

Categorisation of biological and chemical risks according to level of relevance for the EU;

Agreement on the acceptable level of risk;

Setting of priorities, quantifiable targets and performance indicators;

Setting of the amount of resources to be committed to identified threats.

A new Animal Health Strategy for the European Union (2007-2013) where "Prevention is better than cure"

Disease can be devastating on farmers and the economy as a whole – in a specific country, a continent or even globally.

International organisations such as OIE and the World Bank consider Animal Health as a *global public good.* The EU considers the maintenance of "Animal Health Services" in line with international standards (in terms of legislation, structure, organisation, resources, capacities, the role of the private sector and paraprofessionals) as a minimum goal. This is a public investment priority.

Constantly evolving legislation is one of the main mechanisms for EU intervention in animal health, both in the pursuit of Community policy and to implement international obligations. Better regulation principles will be applied through a strengthened partnership and enhanced communication.

The future strategy will aim at replacing the existing series of linked and interrelated policy actions by a single policy framework. The Animal Health Strategy will strive for a single clear regulatory framework converging as far as possible with the OIE/Codex recommendations/standards and guidelines. This regulatory framework will include animal nutrition and animal welfare measures.

The European Commission is responsible for ensuring that unjustified national/ regional rules do not constitute a potential obstacle to the internal market. However, the EU regulatory framework also needs to be suitably flexible to allow for judgements of equivalence, settlements of dispute and efficient responses to changing situations.

Specific attention must be paid to the position of animals kept on a non-commercial basis (i.e. as a hobby) and wildlife, insofar as this impinges on central goals.

Roles and responsibilities will be clearly defined. An incentive-oriented approach is needed at all levels. A revision of the current co-financing instrument is required. More effective procedures will be used for a number of Commission Decisions. The SCFCAH9 will focus on Decisions in which MS and stakeholders have a key interest. Non-regulatory tools must be encouraged as far as possible.

A single horizontal legal framework '! will define and integrate common principles and requirements of existing legislation (intracommunity trade, imports, animal disease control, animal nutrition and animal welfare). Existing legislation will be '! simplified and replaced by this new framework as appropriate, seeking convergence to international standards (OIE/Codex standards) while ensuring a firm commitment to high standards of animal health.

Animal Diseases

Existing compensation schemes are mainly focused on providing a compensation mechanism for animal owners in the event of a disease outbreak. Appropriate sharing of costs, benefits and responsibilities could contribute significantly to the key objectives of the strategy. It could contribute to preventing major financial risks for Member States and the Community by providing incentives for prevention of animal related threats. It would also seek to strengthen Community economic and social cohesion and specifically to reduce the gaps between levels of animal health in the various regions.

On the one hand, Governments have an important role to play in securing our external borders against disease incursions and leading the response to outbreaks of exotic disease. Provision of state compensation is also of utmost importance to compensate for private property destroyed for the public good at least to the extent that the owner is not responsible for the outbreak. In this the protection of public health is a key consideration. On the other hand, responsibility for the health of animals lies primarily with animal owners and collectively with the industry. As a result, animal owners and industry are better placed than others to deal with many of the risks of animal diseases.

There is a clear recognition that the policy needs the full participation and commitment of all parties, including the insurance sector. Ownership of risk is a key issue and new mechanisms must be introduced to involve major stakeholders in decision-making on significant policy issues, in particular for emergency measures. A feasibility study will be necessary to reflect on concrete proposals for the gradual development of an EU harmonised scheme.

Feed Sector

In the feed sector, when large-scale incidents occur, public authorities tend to be heavily burdened with the costs of withdrawal, transport, storage and destruction of feed, food and animals, as well as the costs of analysis and other administrative outlay. Feed business operators are liable for any infringements of the relevant legislation on feed safety and for the direct consequences of the withdrawal from the market, treatment and/ or destruction of any feed, animals and food produced there from.

In 2007, the Commission will submit a report to the European Parliament and the Council setting out the possibilities for an effective system of financial guarantees for feed business operators.

The high level of animal health within the EU will make a key contribution to growth and jobs in Europe by ensuring that farmers and European companies remain competitive and that they have genuine access to the export markets. We need to ensure that European companies, often small and medium-sized enterprises (SMEs), are able to compete fairly in those markets. Unjustified sanitary barriers tend to be increasingly important.

They are complicated, technically challenging and time consuming to detect, analyse and remove. Import conditions for food of animal origin and animal products are largely harmonised. However, this is not the case for exports.

The Commission has exclusive competence for negotiation of bilateral agreements with third countries in the SPS field. For certain third countries, common EU export requirements are specifically defined in bilateral veterinary agreements. Ongoing trade negotiations, in particular the negotiations for Free Trade Agreements with Korea, India and ASEAN include SPS chapters.

The Commission is in a discussion with Member States on the implications of the implementation of existing and future policy on SPS negotiations with third countries in relation to exports. The aim is to ensure respect of the Treaty obligations in relation to the Common Commercial Policy and to present a unified Community approach in negotiations with third countries. The new EU Animal health strategy will contribute to adapt the mix of policy organisations, where appropriate.

Successful biosecurity measures must address isolation of new animals brought to the farm, isolation of sick animals, regulation of the movement of people, animals, and equipment, correct use of feed, and procedures for cleaning and disinfecting facilities. This responsibility lies with the animal owners, including hobby farmers. However, as some contagious pathogens may easily spread from one farm to another a collective approach must be taken in addressing prevention and biosecurity measures.

Effective on-farm biosecurity measures will constitute an important criterion of zoning and compartmentalisation procedures for disease control and/or trade purposes. The EU is the biggest food importer in the world. The Member States' responsibility in border control is to protect the community from potential animal and public health risks arising from international trade of live animals and their products. The challenge is to improve border biosecurity without severely disrupting cross-border movement of people and agricultural goods. In fact, the main safety feature of border controls on declared imports for animal health purposes is the document check, and the EU is dependent upon the accuracy and honesty of the declarations in these documents.

Veterinarians need to work more closely with customs, both at border inspection posts and at points of entry to the Community where goods or animals may enter illegally. There are fundamental questions about: the assessment of risk; trust between national governments; and what can and cannot be accomplished in border inspection facilities and other points of entry (efficiency/effectiveness). On the other hand, it may be difficult for certain developing countries to comply with EU standards and thus engage in trade. The EU should build on ongoing initiatives and improve cooperation with third countries, providing them with technical assistance to help them to satisfy EU animal health requirements for imports and to fight against exotic diseases at source.

Emergency Preparedness

Animal-related emergencies must be dealt with swiftly and effectively using an agreed approach. The possibility for the Commission to take fast-track decisions for emergency action is of high value in limiting and controlling animal-related threats at EU level. In response to ethical concerns and the growing demand for improved animal welfare, the EU has already moved to a more flexible approach to vaccination, as well as improving its policy to control major animal diseases. To decrease the number of animals eliminated will be one of the objectives of the new EU animal health policy (goal 4).

However, different elements make it important that the decision to use vaccination is taken on a case by case basis. Preparation, contingency planning exercises and implementation of emergency preparedness plans are the responsibility of the governments. These plans should be agreed in advance with the cost sharing scheme partners. A key factor in being able to manage an outbreak successfully is knowing where animals and their products are, and controlling their movements.

Animal Testing

The history of animal testing goes back to the writings of the Greeks in the 4th and 3rd centuries BCE, with Aristotle (384-322 BCE) and Erasistratus (304-258 BCE) among the first to perform experiments on living animals. Galen, a physician in 2nd-century Rome, dissected pigs and goats, and is known as the "father of vivisection." Avenzoar, an Arabic physician in 12th-century Moorish Spain who also practiced dissection, introduced animal testing as an experimental method of testing surgical procedures before applying them to human patients.

Basic Science Advances

In 1242, Ibn al-Nafis provided accurate descriptions of the circulation of blood in mammals. A more complete description of this circulation was later provided in the 17th century by William Harvey. In the 18th century, Antoine Lavoisier, used a guinea pig in a calorimetre to prove that respiration was a form of combustion, and Stephen Hales measured blood pressure in the horse. In the 1780s, Luigi Galvani demonstrated that electricity applied to a dead, dissected, frog's leg muscle caused it to twitch, which led to an appreciation for the relationship between electricity and animation. In the 1880s, Louis Pasteur convincingly demonstrated the germ theory of medicine by giving anthrax to sheep. In the 1890s, Ivan Pavlov famously used dogs to describe classical conditioning.

In 1921 Otto Loewi provided the first strong evidence that neuronal communication with target cells occurred via chemical synapses. He extracted two hearts from frogs and left them beating in an ionic bath. He stimulated the attached Vagus nerve of the first heart, and observed its beating slowed. When the second heart was placed in the ionic bath of the first, it also slowed.

In the 1920s, Edgar Adrian formulated the theory of neural communication that the frequency of action potentials, and not the size of the action potentials, was the basis for communicating the magnitude of the signal. His work was performed in an isolated frog nerve-muscle preparation. Adrian was awarded a Nobel Prize for his work.

In the 1960s David Hubel and Torsten Wiesel demonstrated the macrocolumnar organisation of visual areas in cats and monkeys, and provided physiological evidence for the critical period for the development of disparity sensitivity in vision (i.e.: the main cue for depth perception), and were awarded a Nobel Prize for their work.

In 1996 Dolly the sheep was born, the first mammal to be cloned from an adult cell.

Medical Advances

In the 1880s and 1890s, Emil von Behring isolated the diphtheria toxin and demonstrated its effects in guinea pigs. He went on to demonstrate immunity against diphtheria in animals in 1898 by injecting a mix of toxin and antitoxin. This work constituted in part the rationale for awarding von Behring the 1901 Nobel Prize in Physiology and Medicine. Roughly 15 years later, Behring announced such a mix suitable for human immunity which largely banished the diphtheria from the scourges of mankind. The antitoxin is famously commemorated each year in the Iditarod race, which is modelled after the delivery of diphtheria antitoxin to Nome in the 1925 serum run to Nome. The success of the animal studies in producing the diphtheria antitoxin are attributed by some as a cause in the decline of the early 20th century antivivisectionist movement in the USA.

In 1921, Frederick Banting tied up the pancreatic ducts of dogs, and discovered that the isolates of pancreatic secretion could be used to keep dogs with diabetes alive. He followed up these experiments with chemical isolation of insulin in 1922 with John Macleod. These experiments used bovine sources instead of dogs to improve the supply. The first person treated was Leonard Thompson, a 14 year old diabetic who only weighed 65 pounds and was about to slip into a coma and die. After the first dose, the formulation had to be reworked, a process that took 12 days. The second dose was effective. These two won the Nobel Prize in Physiology or Medicine in 1923 for their discovery of insulin and its treatment of diabetes mellitus. Thompson lived 13 more years taking insulin. Before insulin's clinical use, a diagnosis of diabetes mellitus meant death; Thompson had been diagnosed in 1919.

In the 1943, Selman Waksman's laboratory discovered streptomycin using a series of screens to find antibacterial substances from the soil. Waksman coined the term antibiotic with regards to these substances. Waksman would win the Nobel Prize in Medicine in 1952 for his discoveries in antibiotics. Corwin Hinshaw and William Feldman took the streptomycin samples and cured tuberculosis in four guinea pigs with it. Hinshaw followed these studies with human trials that provided a dramatic advance in the ability to stop and reverse the progression of tuberculosis. Mortality from tuberculosis in the UK has diminished from the early 20th century due to better hygiene and improved living standards, but from the moment antibiotics were introduced, the fall became much steeper, so that by the 1980s mortality in developed countries was effectively zero.

In the 1940s, Jonas Salk used Rhesus monkey cross-contamination studies to isolate the three forms of the polio virus that affected hundreds of thousands yearly. Salk's team created a vaccine against the strains of polio in cell cultures of Rhesus monkey kidney cells. The vaccine was made publicly available in 1955, and reduced the incidence of polio 15-fold in the USA over the following five years.

Albert Sabin made a superior "live" vaccine by passing the polio virus through animal hosts, including monkeys. The vaccine was produced for mass consumption in 1963 and is still in use today. It had virtually eradicated polio in the USA by 1965. It has been estimated that 100,000 Rhesus monkeys were killed in the course of developing the polio vaccines, and 65 doses of vaccine were produced for each monkey.

Also in the 1940s, John Cade tested lithium salts in guinea pigs in a search for pharmaceuticals with anticonvulsant properties. The animals seemed calmer in their mood. He then tested lithium on himself, before using it to treat recurrent mania. The introduction of lithium revolutionized the treatment of manic-depressives by the 1970s. Prior to Cade's animal testing, manic-depressives were treated with lobotomy or electro-convulsive therapy.

In the 1950s the first safer, non-volatile anaesthetic halothane was developed through studies on rodents, rabbits, dogs, cats and monkeys. This paved the way for a whole new generation of modern general anaesthetics-also developed by animal studies-without which modern, complex surgical operations would be virtually impossible.

In 1960, Albert Starr pioneered heart valve replacement surgery in humans after a series of surgical advances in dogs. He received the Lasker Medical Award in 2007 for his efforts, along with Alain Carpentier. In 1968 Carpentier made heart valve replacements from the heart valves of pigs, which are pre-treated with gluteraldehyde to blunt immune response. Over 300,000 people receive heart valve replacements derived from Starr and Carpentier's designs annually. Carpentier said of Starr's initial advances "Before his prosthetic, patients with valvular disease would die".

In the 1970s, leprosy multidrug antibiotic treatments were refined using leprosy bacteria grown in armadillos, and were then tested in human clinical trials. Today, the nine-banded armadillo is still used to culture the bacteria that causes leprosy, for studies of the proteomics and genomics (the genome was completed in 1998) of the bacteria, for the purposes of improving therapy and developing vaccines. Leprosy is still prevalent in Brazil, Madagascar, Mozambique, Tanzania, India and Nepal, with over 400,000 cases at the beginning of 2004. The bacteria has not yet been cultured in vitro with success necessary to develop drug treatments or vaccines, and mice and armadillos have been the sources of the bacteria for research.

The non-human primate models of AIDS, using HIV-2, SHIV, and SIV in macaques, have been used as a complement to ongoing research efforts against the virus. The drug tenofovir has had its efficacy and toxicology evaluated in macaques, and found long-term/high-dose treatments had adverse effects not found using short-term/high-dose treatment followed by long-term/low-dose treatment. This finding in macaques was translated into human dosing regimens. Prophylactic treatment with anti-virals has been evaluated in macaques, because introduction of the virus can only be controlled in an animal model. The finding that prophylaxis can be effective at blocking infection has altered the treatment for occupational exposures, such as needle exposures.

Such exposures are now followed rapidly with anti-HIV drugs, and this practice has resulted in measurable transient virus infection similar to the NHP model. Similarly, the mother-to-fetus transmission, and its fetal prophylaxis with antivirals such as tenofovir and AZT, has been evaluated in controlled testing in macaques not possible in humans, and this knowledge has guided antiviral treatment in pregnant mothers with HIV. "The comparison and correlation of results obtained in monkey and human studies is leading to a growing validation and recognition of the relevance of the animal model. Although each animal model has its limitations, carefully designed drug studies in nonhuman primates can continue to advance our scientific knowledge and guide future clinical trials."

Throughout the 20th century, research that used live animals has led to many other medical advances and treatments for human diseases, such as: organ transplant techniques and anti-transplant rejection medications, the heart-lung machine, antibiotics like penicillin, and whooping cough vaccine.

Presently, animal experimentation continues to be used in research that aims to solve medical problems from Alzheimer's disease, multiple sclerosis spinal cord injury, and many more conditions in which there is no useful in vitro model system available.

Treatments to each of the following animal diseases have been derived from animal studies: rabies, anthrax, glanders, Feline immunodeficiency virus (FIV), tuberculosis, Texas cattle fever, Classical swine fever (hog cholera), Heartworm and other parasitic infections.

Basic and applied research in veterinary medicine continues in varied topics, such as searching for improved treatments and vaccines for feline leukemia virus and improving veterinary oncology.

Early Debate

In 1655, physiologist Edmund O'Meara is recorded as saying that "the miserable torture of vivisection places the body in an unnatural state." O'Meara thus expressed one of the chief scientific objections to vivisection: that the pain that the subject endured would interfere with the accuracy of the results.

In 1822, the first animal protection law was enacted in the British parliament, followed by the Cruelty to Animals Act (1876), the first law specifically aimed at regulating animal testing. The legislation was promoted by Charles Darwin, who wrote to Ray Lankester in March 1871:

You ask about my opinion on vivisection. I quite agree that it is justifiable for real investigations on physiology; but not for mere damnable and detestable curiosity. It is a subject which makes me sick with horror, so I will not say another word about it, else I shall not sleep tonight."

Opposition to the use of animals in medical research arose in the United States during the 1860s, when Henry Bergh founded the American Society for the Prevention of Cruelty to Animals (ASPCA), with America's first specifically anti-vivisection organisation being the American AntiVivisection Society (AAVS), founded in 1883.

In the UK, an article in the Medical Times and Gazette on April 28, 1877, indicates that anti-vivisectionist campaigners, mainly clergymen, had prepared a number of posters entitled, "This is vivisection," "This is a living dog," and "This is a living rabbit," depicting animals in a poses that they said copied the work of Elias von Cyon in St. Petersburg, though the article says the images differ from the originals. It states that no more than 10 or a dozen men were actively involved in animal testing on living animals in the UK at that time.

Antivivisectionists of the era generally believed the spread of mercy was the great cause of civilization, and vivisection was cruel. However, in the U.S., the antivivisectionists' efforts were defeated in every legislature, overwhelmed by the superior organisation and influence of the medical community.

The early antivivisectionist movement in the U.S. dwindled greatly in the 1920s, potentially caused by a variety of factors including opposition of the medical community, improvement in medicine through the use of animals, and the tendency of the antivivisectionists to misrepresentation and exaggeration, and their use of inaccurate, vague and outdated references. Overall, this movement had no US legislative success until the passing of the Laboratory Animal Welfare Act, in 1966.

On the other side of the debate, those in favour of animal testing held that experiments on animals were necessary to advance medical and biological knowledge. The founders, in 1831, of the Dublin Zoo—the fourth oldest zoo in Europe, after Vienna, Paris, and London—were members of the medical profession, interested in studying the animals both while they were alive and when they were dead.

Claude Bernard, known as the "prince of vivisectors" and the father of physiology—whose wife, Marie Françoise Martin, founded the first anti-vivisection society in France in 1883—famously wrote in 1865 that "the science of life is a superb and dazzlingly lighted hall which may be reached only by passing through a long and ghastly kitchen." Arguing that "experiments on animals...are entirely conclusive for the toxicology and hygiene of man...the effects of these substances are the same on man as on animals, save for differences in degree," Bernard established animal experimentation as part of the standard scientific method.

In 1896, the physiologist and physician Dr. Walter B. Cannon said "The antivivisectionists are the second of the two types Theodore Roosevelt described when he said, 'Common sense without conscience may lead to crime, but conscience without common sense may lead to folly, which is the handmaiden of crime.'"

These divisions between pro-and anti-animal testing groups first came to public attention during the brown dog affair in the early 20th century, when hundreds of medical students clashed with anti-vivisectionists and police over a memorial to a vivisected dog.

Is Climate Change Increasing Viral Disease in Farm Animals?

Since 1998, there have been increasing outbreaks of the viral disease, bluetongue, among European livestock. Using a newly developed climate-based model that accurately predicts past outbreaks, researchers have provided evidence that climate change is a major driver of these outbreaks.

Bluetongue (BT) is a viral disease of ruminants (which include sheep and cattle) spread by biting midges. For some time it has been widely distributed in Africa, Asia, Australia, South America and North America. Until recently, it was very rare in Europe, but in 1998, an unprecedented series of outbreaks began, causing the deaths of millions of animals and serious economic impacts.

Scientists have proposed that changes in climate may be partly responsible. Furthermore, since it has emerged only recently, scientists believe BT provides a good example for the development of models to describe how climate change may influence diseases in the future.

The study, partly supported by the EU CIRCE project1, developed a framework to evaluate the effects of past and future climate on the risk of the emergence of BT.

The framework integrated climate data into a disease transmission model and evaluated whether the model could reproduce accurately past outbreaks of BT. Good correspondence between the model and historic records suggests that climate was influencing the increase in outbreaks.

Sheep and cattle were considered as these are present in large numbers; data on midge abundance was provided by the Spanish BT national surveillance programme. Past climate data from 1961-2008 was derived from a dataset of observed temperature and rainfall, and future climate data from model simulations provided by ENSEMBLES2 data.

The climate-driven model explained both spatial and temporal variations in the recent emergence and spread of BT in Europe. This included the 2006 BT outbreak in northwest Europe, which occurred in the year that the model predicted the highest risk since at least 1960.

The model also provided insight into the role of drivers in different parts of Europe. For example, in northwest Europe temperature is a major driver of disease risk, whereas in southwest Europe the situation is more complex. In southwest Europe, if rainfall is low then increases in temperature will lead to a decrease in risk of BT outbreaks, and if rainfall increases, higher temperatures will lead to an increase in risk.

The model also quantified the effects of future changes of climate on the risk of BT transmission. Results suggest that by 2050 the number of secondary cases arising from the introduction of one infected animal will increase by 30 per cent in northwest Europe and by 10 per cent in southwest Europe.

The researchers highlighted some weaknesses in the model, such as the lack of species-specific data of the different types of midges, including biting rate, incubation period and mortality rate. They also suggested the data on midge abundance was questionable as it relied on midges caught in light traps, which might not represent the population.

Lastly, there was no accounting for lags in the model which presumes a near-instant impact of changes in climate. Nevertheless, the framework successfully describes past outbreaks of BT in Europe, provides predictions for the future and could be applied to other diseases.

Emerging Animal Diseases and International Trade

Infectious animal and zoonotic diseases are becoming more and more important in the changing farming and trading systems of the industrialised and developing world, writes TheCattleSite Senior Editor, Chris Harris.

Dr. Alejandro A. Schudel from Fundación PROSAIA in Argentina told the World Meat Congress in Cape Town, that some emerging or evolving infectious diseases have the potential to quickly spread from local to international significance, or to jump species barriers-including to humans.

He added that these diseases can have a serious impact on international trade and also in the perception of the consumers with regard to the safety of animal derived products.

"We are facing new challenges in animal diseases," Dr Schudel said.

"In the last 25 years they have spread very quickly and have taken on a global perspective."

He said that there is a significant interaction between both human and animal health now that we face animal and zoonotic diseases of unprecedented magnitude.

He said the world is at the threshold of a new era of emergent and re-emergent diseases that will have a tremendous impact on public health. The significance of its potential consequences has substantially influenced the acceptance of the concept of "Healthy Animals, Safe Food, Healthy People."

Examples of Emerging and Re-Emerging Diseases

Dr Schudel said that this is reflected in the fact that numerous countries have established their own standards and regulations to control diseases.

The effects of globalisation, industrialisation, the restructuring of the agricultural sector, and the growing and sustained demand for animal proteins, are rapidly changing the foundations and the applications of policies directly related to animal health and food safety as well as to the safety of the food supply.

One important aspect is that the increase in diseases is largely in zoonotic diseases-those that can be passed from animal to human.

He estimated that 75 per cent of the emerging diseases are zoonotic.

The factors that influence the spread of disease are environmental, ecological, genetic and political. Poverty and inequality, wars, a lack of domestic political will to tackle disease all influence how it is spread around the world.

Dr Schudel added that this new scenario of worldwide health affects not only the importing and exporting countries, but all countries as a whole, due to the tremendous implications that such events could have on global trade.

The recent outbreaks of Bovine Spongiform Encephalopathy (BSE) in Europe, Asia and North America, the Highly Pathogenic Avian Influenza (HPAI) epidemic that started in South East Asia and the introduction of Foot and Mouth (FMD) disease in Europe, are typical examples of this new scenario.

The quick detection of these emerging, re-emerging and zoonotic diseases and the consequent reaction will be the decisive factor in order to be able to quickly overcome the threat posed by such events.

He said that the lessons learned from the outbreaks of these diseases were that there was an increased need for food safety measures, increased communication to the consumer and there was a raised awareness among the general public of issues of animal welfare and well being.

He added that the impact of the diseases was felt by everyone-rich and poor alike and that there was a serious financial consequence to any outbreak of disease. The 2001 UK foot and mouth disease outbreak had a financial impact of £13 billion. In the US it has been estimated that the financial costs of an outbreak of foot and mouth disease would be between $7 billion and $14 billion. The cost of the avian influenza outbreak in Asia has already been estimated at between $8 billion and $12 billion.

Animal health has a lot to do with food safety and healthy animals have a lot to do with safe food he said.

The readiness of any country to face an animal emerging disease, and its capacity to respond, depend in great measure to the preparedness of its Veterinary Services.

The lack of infrastructures which support diagnostic laboratories, veterinarians, expert services and worldwide vigilance, are insufficient, and this fact is clearly seen among developed and developing nations.

He said there is an urgent need to improve veterinary services and a need for transparent veterinary services.

Another extremely important aspect that needs to be addressed is the quick and efficient manner on how to alert the consumer about the scientific based risks of these diseases with regards to food safety.

He said that the outbreaks of BSE and Avian Influenza are cases that show the need for transparency and swift communication.

Animal Health authorities and Public Health authorities have to confront the issues in a coordinated manner.

International organisations are bringing about joint efforts, and the World Organisation for Animal Health (OIE) has clearly said it should play a role when facing the difficulties that these diseases pose on a worldwide level.

Effective global security can only be achieved if all trading countries comply with the internationally agreed upon standards and guidelines, effectively training people in the industry and ensuring the availability of adequate human and material veterinary resources and he also called for a strong global quality certification process to verify the integrity of products and the health of animals.

Many countries share a common concern about the emergence of animal diseases and zoonosis or the deliberate misuse of pathogenic biological agents that could affect the public health as well as food and animal production.

Existing methods of disease prevention and containment regulations as well as international guidelines and standards are available and should be followed in order to procure early detection and a quick containment, Dr Schudel said.

Predicting Changes for Parasite and Vector Induced Animal Diseases

Climate change could have a major influence on animal health, both directly and indirectly, by affecting the parasites and vectors that spread diseases, according to Eric Hoberg, an Agricultural Research Service (ARS) zoologist at the Agricultural Research Centre in Beltsville.

Climate change can alter an animal's relationship with parasites and vectors. These changes can influence where parasites and vectors thrive, making certain geographical regions more or less amenable to them. Climate change can also alter when and for how long parasites and vectors pose a threat to agricultural animals. Climate can determine how pathogens are distributed, transmitted and evolve, and can influence the factors associated with emerging disease and how animals respond to those diseases. Significant environmental changes have been well documented in recent decades, and some of these changes are causing trouble for livestock.

Dr Eric Hoberg is one of many ARS scientists investigating the probable impact of climate changes on agricultural parasites and virus vectors. Their research is generating information that could help producers prepare for and respond to heightened disease threats.

In one study, Dr Hoberg collaborated with several Canadian scientists to investigate the influence of climate change on parasitic lungworms known as *Protostrongylus stilesi* in Arctic mammals. Although the lungworms had never before been observed in muskoxen, the scientists observed them in muskoxen that share habitat with Dall's sheep. Environmental changes that bring the two animals into contact more frequently could result in larger parasite populations.

"Climate change alters the boundaries between different species and between natural and managed lands," Dr Hoberg says. "When these boundaries break down, it becomes possible for pathogens to switch between hosts."

Muskoxen are not a major agricultural animal in the United States, but their interaction with lungworms and Dall's sheep could be used to establish predictive models that could help US animal producers better understand how pathogens switch between hosts. Climate change may also influence insects that spread diseases. At the ARS Arthropod-Borne Animal Diseases Research Laboratory (ABADRL) in Laramie, Wyoming, scientists are investigating several vectored diseases, including bluetongue and Rift Valley fever (RVF).

"In recent years we've seen an incursion of bluetongue virus in Europe, but whether that's affected by climate change or not hasn't yet been determined," says ABADRL microbiologist, Bill Wilson.

Muskoxen

Several factors influenced by climate change could explain the spread of bluetongue virus, says ABADRL entomologist, Kristine Bennett. Higher temperatures could enable *Culicoides imicola*, the disease's primary vector in Europe, to inhabit a much larger geographic area. Higher temperatures could enhance viral replication, potentially enabling indigenous Culicoides populations to vector the disease. And warmer winter temperatures could enable more Culicoides to survive the winter, extending their influence.

Other factors are at play in the case of RVF, a viral disease that occurs in Africa and recently has spread beyond the continent's borders into the Arabian Peninsula.

"RVF outbreaks are closely connected to cycling global climate variability caused by El Niño Southern Oscillation phenomena – particularly rainfall and flooding, which introduce the virus into livestock populations by facilitating the hatching of virus-infected mosquito eggs resting in the soil," says Ken Linthicum, director of the ARS Centre for Medical, Agricultural and Veterinary Entomology in Gainesville, Florida.

"Our research hasn't focused on climate trends, but we do know that elevated sea surface temperatures, such as those associated with El Niño cycles, are related to heavy rainfall and flooding, which are related to RVF outbreaks," Dr Linthicum says.

Dr Linthicum led a team of scientists in developing a model that in 2006 successfully predicted an RVF outbreak in Africa several months before the outbreak occurred. This early warning enabled international aid organisations to increase disease surveillance and to conduct public information, animal vaccine and insect control programs. Since then, the model has predicted outbreaks in southern Africa, Sudan and the Horn of Africa. Tools like this could be essential for early detection and control of RVF, should it ever enter the United

States. Since the 1950s, ocean buoys and satellite instrument monitors have clearly documented increasing surface temperatures in the Indian Ocean. Dr Linthicum and his colleagues believe these rising temperatures and related rainfall result in more frequent, smaller outbreaks of RVF.

"When large outbreaks do occur, they tend to be bigger and more widespread than those we observed in the past," he says. This information could help policymakers mobilise outbreak response efforts.

"The potential effects of climate change are not yet fully understood," says ARS national programme leader, Cyril Gay. "But evidence suggests that animal health could be affected by rising ambient and ocean temperatures. To protect US livestock from parasite and vector-borne diseases, scientists must be engaged in research on many fronts."

Regular surveillance will provide up-to-date information about changes in pathogen populations. Laboratory and field research will help illuminate how climate changes influence pathogen characteristics, and models will help researchers and producers predict and plan for pathogen threats. With a nationwide network of research facilities and a history of groundbreaking pathogen research, ARS is well positioned to provide research, expertise and tools to address any parasite or vector-borne disease threats that arise in response to a changing global climate.

Animal Welfare Guidelines for Beef Cattle Farms

There is a significant body of national and EU legislation enacted relating to animal welfare. Here, the Irish Agriculture and Food Development Authority explain how compliance with welfare legislation is an important requirement for the National Beef Assurance Scheme and the Code of Good Farming Practice.

Introduction

Many retailers and major food service chains will only purchase Irish beef that originates from assured farms. Animal welfare standards are a prominent feature of Irish and European farm assurance schemes.

The welfare of farm animals is an increasingly important issue for the Irish beef industry. Research studies conducted by the Teagasc National Food Centre (NFC) and various other researchers indicate that both domestic and foreign consumers of Irish beef are becoming more conscious of animal welfare issues. The NFC studies suggest that consumers may also view high animal welfare standards as an indicator that food is safe, healthier and of high quality. Thus, perception of animal welfare standards can affect the consumers' image of Irish beef.

Good animal welfare has always being an integral part of the husbandry content of Irish livestock production systems.

Irish beef production systems are grass based and extensive by nature. Nonetheless, there are aspects of beef cattle production such as the housing of animals during winter, castration, dehorning, transport, handling and slaughter that have the potential to cause stress, pain and injury if not managed correctly.

This booklet briefly summarises key animal welfare standards and best farm assurance practice that producers should be able to demonstrate to other stakeholders in the food chain.

The appendices detail sources of relevant animal welfare legislation.

The Five Freedoms Concept

In essence an animal welfare Code of Practice is the application of sensible and sensitive animal husbandry practices to the livestock present on the farm. Animal welfare is concerned with the well-being of the animal and complements the objectives of beef assurance schemes that demonstrate the production of safe beef to consumers and food chain stakeholders.

Welfare codes usually list five basic freedoms that should underpin on farm animal welfare best practice. The five freedoms are listed below and provides an overall concept of animal welfare. One-freedom from thirst, hunger and malnutrition Two-freedom from discomfort Three-freedom from pain, injury and disease Four-freedom to express normal patterns of behaviour Five-freedom from fear and distress

Welfare Guidelines

Stockman

Stockmanship is a key factor in animal welfare. The stockman should have training and or the necessary experience in cattle husbandry. Without competent diligent stockmanship animal welfare will be compromised.

A competent stockman should be able to:

- recognise whether or not the animals are in good health (signs of ill health include: loss of appetite, listlessness, cessation of cudding, discharge from eyes or nostrils, dribbling, persistent coughing, lameness, swollen joints, scouring, rapid loss of condition or emaciation, excessive scratching, abnormal skin conditions or other unusual conditions)

- understand the significance of a change in the behaviour of the animals
- know when veterinary treatment is required
- implement a planned herd health programme (e.g. preventative treatments, vaccination programmes if necessary)
- implement appropriate animal feeding and grassland management programmes
- recognise if the general environment (indoors or outdoors) is adequate for the promotion of good health and welfare
- have management skills appropriate to the scale and technical requirements of the production system
- handle animals with care, avoiding undue stress.

A good stockman will individually inspect all animals at least once per day. Particular categories of animals will require more frequent inspection e.g. young calves or cows in late pregnancy etc. Formal training and/or experience working under the supervision of a competent stockman is strongly recommended where inexperienced persons are taking over responsibility for animal husbandry on a farm.

Common veterinary type activities (e.g. dosing, injecting, castration) should not be attempted without direct appropriate supervision until the stockman is competent to carry out these activities. People already involved in animal management/husbandry should keep themselves updated in technological developments that can prevent or correct welfare problems.

Husbandry Practices and Relevant Records

Husbandry practices should minimise stress to the animal. All farms must have proper animal handling facilities including pens and a crush where an animal can be restrained with minimum risk of injury or stress. Good handling facilities also benefit the safety of the personnel involved in handling the animals.

Early and frequent contact with competent persons particularly at an early age greatly reduces the stress to animals subsequently.

Cattle are gregarious animals who will socialise with each other, when young calves are individually penned they should be able to see other calves.

Many assurance schemes and regulatory requirements require that key records are maintained on the farm. Some of these records help producers to demonstrate that best practice has been implemented in relation to animal health and welfare standards. Key records include:

- Bovine Herd Register
- Animal Remedies Record
- Animal Feed Records.

Some assurance schemes also require producers to maintain a Planned Herd Health Programme Checklist. Some retailer assurance schemes also require producers to document recommended operating procedures in the event of an emergency (fire in a livestock shed, operational guidelines for replacement stockperson in the event that the stockperson is away)

Basic Farm Biosecurity

Producers are advised to follow good on-farm biosecurity measures to protect their livestock and crops from the constant threat of pests and diseases. Biosecurity Queensland principal veterinary officer Janet Berry said being aware of biosecurity meant keeping animals safe from disease and ensuring continued market access for produce.

"Straightforward measures built into everyday practice will go a long way toward protecting your farm and your future," she said.

"Animal owners should assess the risks to their animals and act to reduce the risks."

Purchased Livestock

The movement of new animals onto your property represents the highest risk of introducing disease into your herd or flock. Inspect the animals carefully for disease before buying them.

Always request the history and supporting paperwork, such as the vendor declaration or national health statement, before you buy the animals. Isolate new animals to make sure they are disease and weed free before mixing with your stock.

Stray Animals

Poor fencing can allow stray livestock, and wild or feral animals to mix with your stock and introduce disease. Keep all gates shut and check fences regularly.

People

People can carry animal pests and diseases. Ask all visitors where they have been previously; whether they've had contact with other animals, or been abroad and possibly brought diseases home. Keep a register of all visitors.

Restrict visitor access to your property and make sure they don't go near animals unless they have clean clothes and have disinfected hands and footwear.

Vehicles and Equipment

Vehicles and equipment can carry pests and diseases. Control the entry of vehicles onto the property and ensure they stay in a designated vehicle area. Use your own vehicles to transport visitors or material around the farm.

Maintain clean and disinfected equipment and do not share with other animal owners.

Feed and Water

Feed and water can contain pests and diseases. Always request a commodity vendor declaration with purchased feed. Keep feed in a clean dry storage area and ensure it does not become mouldy. Make sure that water sources are not contaminated by wild or feral animals or birds.

Dr Berry said there were major outcomes of having farm biosecurity plans in place.

"Outcomes include improved profitability through the reduction of diseases, less need for expensive chemical treatments or vaccinations and improved animal production," she said.

"Farm biosecurity plans can reduce the risk of introducing pests and diseases onto a property that are already present on your neighbours farm or elsewhere.

"Good planning now will also reduce the impact of the next disease emergency.

"The rapid and wide geographical spread of emergency diseases can be controlled more easily if all livestock owners begin to practice farm biosecurity now."

Global Approaches to Farm Animal Welfare

This article is taken from the proceedings of the Livestock Care Conference, held by Alberta Farm Animal Care. New emphasis on animal welfare in the U.S., Europe and internationally is changing the dynamics of how food is produced and marketed worldwide.

For those still not convinced that consumer concerns over animal welfare represent anything more than a fringe mentality, consider the following: according to a 2007 American Farm Bureau survey, 68 percent of Americans polled think the government should take an active role in promoting the welfare of farm animals.

Nothing new, right? Most producers have heard statistics like this before, but there are two things that set this one apart. First, it's the result of a poll conducted by an independent grassroots farm agency rather than a group, such as People for the Ethical Treatment of Animals (PETA), with a specific agenda on animal welfare. Secondly, it's a call for government intervention in a country that typically waves the flag for government that is as small as possible.

To Dr. Ed Pajor, director for the Centre for Animal Well-Being at Purdue University in Indiana, it's an example of a new social ethic concerning animals – and one that has turned long-relied-upon models of livestock production and marketing on their heads.

Pajor spent two years studying the animal welfare culture of Europe and the United States – two markets with far different approaches to animal welfare that are nevertheless heading toward a similar end-point. In a presentation at the Livestock Care Conference in Red Deer, Alberta April 4, he offered an overview of his findings and what they may mean to the Canadian livestock industry going forward. "Emerging animal welfare policy from powerful world bodies such as the World Organisation for Animal Health (OIE) is set to have a major influence on policy in North America," he says. "Meanwhile, the free market is already having a major impact, with major food companies increasingly preferring to work with suppliers who can provide proof of responsible animal welfare practices.

"This means higher expectations for the livestock industry, but it can also mean a great opportunity for those who can provide this assurance. The bottom line is that demand for transparent animal welfare will not be going away. It's a reflection of a whole new way in which society views animals, and is quickly becoming part of the culture of agriculture as well."

The OIE Animal-centred Approach

No discussion of farm animal welfare at the global level would be complete without mentioning the World Organisation for Animal

Health, otherwise known as the OIE. Created in 1924 to develop standards to combat the outbreak of animal diseases, OIE standards have become the international reference in the field of animal diseases for the World Trade Organisation (WTO). In recent years, this relationship has helped the OIE become a key developer of international standards for animal welfare as well.

Countries are under no obligation to adopt OIE standards and guidelines, says Pajor. However, the OIE's emphasis on science-based guidelines and its "five freedoms" of animal care (freedom from hunger and thirst; freedom from discomfort; freedom from pain, injury and disease; freedom to express normal behaviour; and freedom from fear and distress) have made the organisation a standard-bearer for countries seeking approaches that satisfy customer demands.

"What sets the OIE's guidelines apart is its emphasis on animal-based criteria as opposed to resource-based criteria. The difference is that the former sets out easily-measurable guidelines related to design and inputs such as space allowances, temperature ranges, and air quality. Animal-based criteria, on the other hand, focuses on performance and output factors such as survival rate, disease and injury, behaviour, and reaction to handlers. These criteria are very difficult to measure, but they address the needs of individual animals much more comprehensively."

Speaking in a general sense, Europe is different culturally from countries such as the U.S. in that its citizens look to government for a comprehensive degree of leadership, says Pajor. And, true to the wishes of its populace, Europe took a lead on animal welfare in the 1960s, when the Council of Europe began to focus on animal welfare issues.

Today, animal welfare has become part of Europe's culture of agriculture. The European model of developing animal welfare law follows the top-down model of the OIE – albeit on a more prescriptive basis – by providing guidelines and minimum requirements that often become law at the national level.

The Council of Europe, which includes 46 member states, issues both binding conventions and non-binding guidelines on animal care for its members. The 27 countries that make up the European Union also fall under directives established by the EU-27, he says. These directives, which are almost always based on reports from scientific experts, generally focus on animal-centred outcomes such as space allowance per animal, freedom of movement, social interaction and the limitation of painful interventions.

In addition to government-driven legislation and standards, animal welfare also plays a large role in industry-based quality assurance schemes. “Industry-driven quality assurance is considered very important to European consumers, especially niche markets, and are often stricter than other regulations,” says Pajor.

Although much of the above may sound very prescriptive, the fact is that Europe has based most of its animal welfare activity on the wishes of European consumers. They are able to do so because of a strong foundation of data measuring public opinion – a tool that is largely missing in North America, says Pajor.

“The Eurobarometre, a series of surveys on the attitudes of Europeans on a variety of topics, breaks opinion on animal welfare issues down by individual countries. Not surprisingly, these opinions vary in the same way they might vary between, for example, Calgary and Toronto. The overall message, however, is that, to Europeans as a whole, animal welfare is considered an important attribute of overall food quality.”

This infrastructure of public opinion is helping to drive the Welfare Quality Project, a $27 million effort involving 17 countries and 44 universities and institute which stands to become the next generation of animal welfare in Europe. One of the key goals of the project is to develop criteria which capture the public's description of animal welfare.

“I believe this project will have a significant impact on North American agriculture,” says Pajor. “It won't reflect just a few people's opinion – it will be the opinion of a lot of people in a lot of countries with a lot of scientific power backing it up.”

Animal Welfare: Driven by Economics

In the U.S., it's been the private sector that has taken the lead on animal welfare activity, with Burger King's decision to discontinue the acceptance of hogs raised in gestation stalls being one of the most prominent examples. “For the most part, however, animal welfare in the U.S. is based on voluntary guidelines, although state bans on specific production systems are appearing and animal law is becoming a rapidly growing area of law,” says Pajor.

Animal welfare is being built into several private sector-based quality assurance strategies in the U.S. However, Pajor says there is a general tendency to emphasize resource or engineering-based criteria over the kind of animal-focused criteria modelled by the OIE. This approach may not be enough moving forward, however.

"A recent Gallup poll showed that 71 percent of respondents felt that animals deserved some protection, while 25 percent felt that they deserved the same rights as people," says Pajor. "Twenty-five percent is a huge number. And while it's possible that many respondents had companion animals in mind when forming these results, there are implications here on how they think about other types of animals as well. The fact that the same poll showed that 62 percent of respondents favoured passing strict laws concerning the treatment of farm animals bears this out."

Pajor believes consumers, often informed by activists, will continue to play a role in industry action on animal welfare. "By targeting just a few firms, activists are achieving de facto changes in industry regulations in the U.S. These regulations are not imposed by legislators, but by firms seeking a competitive advantage. If you can convince Wal-Mart that animals should be produced in a certain way, there will be a huge impact on how they're produced."

Where We're Headed?

The bottom line, says Pajor, is that animal welfare is here to stay, with guidelines and standards continuing to be developed at all levels, including international agreements and multinational companies. A key strategy moving forward, he says, will be to bullet-proof animal welfare assurance programs against external criticism as much as possible.

"These processes will need to be as transparent as possible, complete with third party audits. Having codes without assessment, audit and teeth is something that will come under more and more criticism."

The livestock industry can also expect animal welfare expectations to become more animal-centred, he says. "We will have more and more undercover video of operations that have been certified. If assurance programs are not taken seriously, consumers will lose trust in our systems and the public has limited trust already. If animal welfare is not embraced wholeheartedly as a necessary element of animal production, grassroots efforts will fall apart and be filled by legislation."

Animal Science-Recent Progress and Future Challenges

The goal of animal science remains efficient animal production according to Professor John Oldham, reports editor, Jackie Linden, for The Cattle Site.

Professor John Oldham of Scottish Agricultural Colleges in Edinburgh was invited to give the Hammond Lecture by the British Society of Animal Science (BSAS) at its annual meeting in Belfast this year. He discussed the developments and understanding brôught by previous generations of animal scientists, including Sir John Hammond, in whose memory the opening lecture of the BSAS is dedicated, and how these studies remain just as important today to feed a growing world population at a time of climate change.

Animal science spans a broad compass, Professor Oldham said. It tends to be considered as a study of animals (nature, function, productivity etc) that are under the management of Man in some way. This differentiates it from zoology, excludes wildlife and provides boundaries with at last some aspects of veterinary and biomedical sciences that can be rather indistinct. It covers both the understanding of animals as biological systems and the role of animals as components of broader systems.

"By being allied to animals that are under management, I take it as implicit that any consideration of progress in animal science needs to include not only progress in intellectual understanding but also progress in the utility of that understanding in practice. This does not deny the value of animals to animal science to inform broader biological understanding," said Professor Oldham.

There has been considerable scientific effort and increases in understanding, both on animals themselves and on their roles in systems, although rather more in the former than in the latter, he explained. Equally, there are future challenges both at the level of the animal as a phenotype and for animals in systems of management, In each case, the great challenge is not simply to understand the behaviour – in the broadest sense – of the animal or system, but also to predict it.

'Recent' is a word that is open to some interpretation. The rate at which some new techniques cna help to generate data in research can make it appear that rates of progress are accelerating. 'Recent' progress in such areas might be considered to span small numbers of years. But a broader perspective is needed to recognise some of the major areas of progress.

Progress in any science is driven by a mixture of imagination to generate the ideas that are worth pursuing, and the acquisition of appropriate techniques to allow those ideas to be tested. Sir John Hammond was a fount of ideas on reproduction, growth and development in the inter-war years and through the 1950s. His insights and techniques led the way in practical improvements in reproduction and his concepts of growth and development have generally stood the tests of time. Like Hammond's waves of growth, progress in animal science has been influenced by waves of technical development. Professor Oldham cited the eamples of the advent of chromatographic techniques in the early post-war years allowed access to rapid analytical methods that underpinned progress in nutrition and physiology especially.

Isotropic tracing techniques gave access to more quantitative understanding of metabolism as well as facilitating analysis. More recently, molecular techniques have opened avenues to understanding that were previously closed. And advance in computational and statistical techniques have not only supported the rapid delivery of thoer methods but have also allowed the realisation of ideas that, in some areas – especially genetics – were formed a significant time ago but were inaccessible for want of computational power.

Progress in genetics has helped to develop animals whose rates of productivity are dramatically increased although sometimes with negative associated consequences – which are now being corrected by adjustments to selection approaches, Professor Oldham said. The promise of molecular approaches to replace more conventional quantitative methods has not yet been fully realised, although the prospects of using genome-wide selection are considerable. Understanding of nutrition and nutritional biochemistry has yielded rationing schemes that work tolerably well and allow some control over the qualities of products that animals produce. Our understanding of reproductive processes has grown substantially, but too often the application of new knowledge has been in the 'catch-up' mode, aiming to correct problems introduced by other 'advances'.

Research on pregnancy and lactation for all mammalian species, including our own, has though, been considerably advanced through the animal sciences. Our understanding of the processes of disease have been enabled through the animal as well as the veterinary and meical sciences, and increasingly, methods of control can be expected to include broad-based approaches that will call on the products of a range of animal sciences. The welfare of animals, as sentient beings, is better appreciated and open to assessment and improvement. But the prediction of phenotypic expression – what an animal will actually do given a knowledge of its genotype and its environment – is still as aspiration rather than a reality.

Professor Oldham said that, on broader knowledge fronts, the impacts of animals on their environment are better understood now than they were. Management of waste to reduce pollution or grazing to achieve biodiversity goals is more possible. Animals also influence the social or operating environments. For example, systems of animal management can be important fro social cohesion and are important sources of work power or equity.

The impacts of animals on the environment are a source of much current concern, though, he said. Some of this relates to issues around climate change, others to the management of pollution or of managing biodiversity. Yet other concerns are to do with perceived negative contributions of animal products to the healthiness of the human diet, At the same time, the growing size of the human population and its ability to afford moe animal products in the global diet has increased, and it likely to continue to increase, the global demands for animals and their products.

This is the big driver that creates the grand challenges for animal sciences to address, Professor Oldham emphasised. The need is to produce animal products in appropriate abundance that are beneficial (or at worst, not detrimental) to the healthiness of our diets, that are produced with minimal waste, (by efficient use of resources and minimisation of losses through disease and reproductive failure especially), no negative impacts on, and preferably benefits to, the environment and in socially acceptable ways.

He said: "To achieve these results, if such is possible, I would expect to see the next stages of progress in the animal sciences being more integrative and predictive. Synthesis of understanding to enable the prediction of functional behaviour of animals as systems and animals in systems (and the behaviour of those systems) as well as continuing lines of discovery to enable this to happen should be to the fore."

A sharp eye on the outcome, and not simply the understanding, is merited. Sir John Hammond was an outstanding scientist – but his goal as science to enable efficient animal production, and we still need that, Professor Oldham concluded.

Learning & Profiting from Animal Welfare Trends

England's largest supermarket paying dairy farmers 15 to 20 percent more to improve welfare. McDonald's leading the way with higher livestock welfare standards. Farmers worldwide taking steps to integrate welfare into quality assurance schemes.

These developments are signals of monumental shifts in expectations and approaches surrounding animal welfare, each with major implications for the livestock industry.

Helping make sense of the trends and what they mean for producers both in Europe and North America was Dr. John Webster of the University of Bristol in England, who delivered a presentation on the subject at the Livestock Care Conference, April 4 in Red Deer. The conference was hosted by Alberta Farm Animal Care (AFAC), a partnership of Alberta's major livestock groups with a mandate to promote responsible, humane animal care within the livestock industry.

"We have reached a pivotal time in animal welfare," says Webster. "This includes many changes and challenges. But for the livestock industry, the good news is that it also includes profit-generating opportunities for farmers related to producing a value added product, which are critical to their survival in a competitive environment."

This assessment and the details that support it mean a lot coming from Webster. One of the world's leading authorities on animal welfare issues, Webster was a founding member of the UK Farm Animal Welfare Council and is the original proponent of the "five freedoms" concept that has become central to emerging animal welfare policy and strategies worldwide. While he sees that animal agriculture still has substantial room to improve when it comes to implementing systems of continual welfare improvement, strong progress is being made and innovations are gaining steam in many countries, particularly in Europe but also in North America.

"I wouldn't want to fool anyone by saying all steps to improve animal welfare will improve profitability for livestock producers," says Webster. "But the way things are moving, I would say to the livestock industry that being self protective and saying there's nothing wrong is not your best solution. There is an opportunity there in terms of value-added products. Just think: if we can do it better, they're very likely to pay us."

What is Welfare Science?

New Definitions, New Expectations

Critical to understanding the new trends in animal welfare is understanding the concept of welfare itself, says Webster. This is important not only to society in general and to the livestock industry, but also to the growing ranks of 'welfare scientists' who will play an essential role in the ongoing development of welfare standards.

In this context, the traditional questions and concepts related to welfare have undergone a major updating, he argues.

For example, the typical questions traditionally posed by welfare scientists to assess animal welfare are today inadequate. These include questions such as: Is the animal living a normal life? Is the animal fit and healthy? How does the animal feel?

"If the first question was adequate, we would be saying all swine should live in the woods. If the second was adequate, we'd be fine with gestation crates so long as the animal was healthy. The third question is probably the closest to being useful, but is still not quite refined enough to provide a comprehensive assessment of welfare."

For a modern definition, Webster supports one derived and extended from earlier definitions by Dr. David Fraser of the University of British Columbia and Donald Broom of Cambridge University. This definition states that animal welfare is "The physical and mental state of a sentient animal (one sensitive in perception or and feelings) as it seeks to cope with environmental challenge."

"Welfare then doesn't just mean feeling good," says Webster. "It is the full spectrum from feeling very good to genuine suffering. And it is defined by both its physical and emotional state."

The concept of sentience is key to the definition, he notes. In pending European Community legislation, farm animals are recognised as sentient creatures.

"This reinforces that farm animals are not simply commodities. They are sentient creatures and we must respect their sentience." Webster makes a distinction between animal welfare and animal well-being. Animal welfare, he says, covers the full spectrum of animal feeling. Animal well-being, on the other hand is defined by an ability to have sustained mental and physical health, to avoid suffering and to generally feel good about life.

"For farm animals, this would include things like comfort, companionship and security, which are particularly important to animals in a herd species," says Webster.

The aspiration for those looking after farm animals, he suggests, should be to promote a sense of well-being within the context of a healthy agricultural industry. This aspiration may not be practical to achieve all the time, but the goal should be to realise it "as much as possible" and to continually strive for improvement

A Sentient View of the World

Feelings that Matter

Sentience itself too, requires an updated definition in the context of animal welfare, says Webster, suggesting that a useful definition is "feelings that matter."

A sentient animal will interpret stimuli at three levels, he explains. These include a basic reflex level, a second emotional level achieved by all sentient animals and a third cognitive level achieved by humans and to some degree by most sentient animals.

Sentient animals do not just live in the present, he says. They are motivated, by emotion and cognition, to action. "The strength of motivation to action is a measure of how important these things are to them."

This concept is a foundation for an increasing number of new studies in animal welfare, which study animal responses to stressors and other stimuli as a means of validating issues of animal pain and suffering and also of gauging their relative importance to animal welfare and well-being.

Earlier pioneering studies in this vein have shown, for example, that animals will self-medicate and perform similar coping actions in response to various negative stimuli.

"If the coping action is successful, the sentient animal with cognitive capacity will learn from it and repeat it under the same circumstance," says Webster. "This is evidence of a highly sentient animal.

The Cost of Coping

From an animal science point of view, Webster suggests the best studies today are those that recognise the "cost of coping" for an animal rather than simply an alarm response, since some animals may not respond greatly if they have learned the "cost" of doing so is not worthwhile or not effective. "It's much more useful to measure the stress-specific cost of coping."

This leads to a definition of suffering, notes Webster, which he defines as a state where an animal cannot cope, or has extreme difficulty coping with a stressor. "This occurs when the stressor is too prolonged or simply too much, or because the animal is unable to respond in a way that will improve how it feels." Examples he says are swine in gestation stalls or hens in battery cages, which are unable to respond in a way that will improve their condition.

Awareness of this is key to recognising welfare issues and seeking improvements, he says.

"The old way of thinking is that animals can experience pain, but that is just about it. Today we increasingly recognise that suffering is much more than just pain and that animals have this broader capacity to suffer." They also have strong capacity for a higher quality of life, to which those responsible for animals must aspire.

The bottom line of the new definitions and thinking on welfare is that expectations are rising, says Webster. "Suffering and pleasure are defined by the capacity to feel, not the capacity to think. And we cannot assume that the capacity to feel is proportional to intelligence, as we define it." This brings animals on more of a level plane to humans in terms of what society considers acceptable in terms of being subject to pain and suffering.

Marketplace Driving New Systems

For the livestock industry, this means expectations for how farm animals are treated are also continuing to rise. "We recognise that farm animals are sentient and have capacity to suffer," says Webster. "This raises the bar for our responsibility in taking care of these animals."

While legislation for improving welfare has been relatively slow to reflect these new expectations, the free market, operating through the likes of McDonald's and other major food retailers is having a major impact.

As a result, animal welfare is increasingly being viewed as an important component of emerging quality assurance schemes. "Increasingly and inevitably in Europe now, quality assurance schemes are including criteria for assessment of animal welfare," says Webster. "And if animal welfare is not up to the standards of the scheme, the farmer will be lost from the scheme. Many of these schemes are driven by supermarkets and big retailers who are marketing their products on a high welfare platform because consumers are making choices based on that platform."

Webster portrayed new expectations as moving toward a "virtuous bicycle" model, where incorporating welfare standards as part of food quality assurance can deliver benefits to all parts of a "fork-to-farm" market-driven chain, including animals, producers and consumers."

The front wheel of the bicycle includes a system for monitoring animal welfare, he explains. The back wheel is a public component that includes a review and feedback to the producer "This model will probably be based on an animal-based, external assessment leading to a constant cycle of action and review to achieve a state of steady improvement of animal welfare," says Webster.

"At the moment, this is not really happening. There are monitoring systems, some of them are quite good, but they're not yet leading to action. With time, they will."

Fast-changing Times

As the marketplace leads the way, policy and regulation is also making headway, he says.

Ideas developed by Webster such as the Five Freedoms are now being taken up in Europe in a big way and are expected to become European standards within the decade.

This will place pressure on North America to adopt similar approaches.

"What we're heading towards is an environment where the marketplace expects high welfare but also expects to pay more to those who supply that high welfare."

If Europe is an indication, trends are moving quickly, he observes. And pressure is not just on livestock producers to adjust but on the food system as a whole.

In one recent development, the UK's largest food retailer, the Waitrose supermarket chain, introduced a high welfare scheme that included granting five year contracts to dairy producers that included a 15 to 20 percent increase in the price of milk.

"The public perception was that producers couldn't improve welfare because the supermarkets were not paying them enough and that led to the scheme," says Webster. "That's something we wouldn't have seen happen 10 years ago."

Advances in Immunology-The Best Shot at Disease Prevention

That was the year officials at the U.S. Centres for Disease Control and Prevention declared the elimination of rubella in the United States.

The eradication of this and other devastating human diseases, such as polio and smallpox, has been due largely to vaccine development and aggressive immunisation programs. Today, vaccines have minimised the toll of many pernicious diseases that used to devastate human health, and animals have benefited too.

In the last century, scientists in the Agricultural Research Service (ARS) developed vaccines that helped eradicate hog cholera, which once cost the U.S. swine industry tens of millions of dollars every year. ARS researchers have also developed vaccines for other animal diseases, such as Marek's disease in chickens and enteric septicemia in catfish, reducing animal suffering and enabling the United States to develop one of the world's safest and most efficient animal production systems.

ARS scientists continue to advance the fields of immunology and vaccinology today, with research into the mechanisms pathogens use to evade the immune system and discovering pathways that will lead to protective immunity and disease resistance. Researchers have also been instrumental in helping to develop a universal toolkit—comprised of species-specific immunological reagents—to gauge immune responses in agricultural animals.

As recently as five years ago, such tools were flawed or nonexistent. But following the 2003 ARS Immunology Research Workshop, scientists stepped up efforts to develop immune toolkits for agricultural animals.

"At the workshop we established networks, both national and international, to identify the most significant toolkit needs for different species," says National Program Leader Cyril Gay.

The U.S. Veterinary Immune Reagent Network was established to develop these toolkits. With a $2.15 million grant from the U.S. Department of Agriculture's Cooperative State Research, Education and Extension Service, the network has started work on five species: cattle, horses, poultry, swine and fish. Two ARS researchers, Hyun Lillehoj and Joan Lunney, are chairing the chicken and swine efforts, respectively.

The network, whose researchers hail from a variety of government, university and institutional organisations, has made significant progress, and researchers are already in the early stages of developing monoclonal antibodies for use in animal disease and vaccination studies.

Within the United States, more than 1,300 vaccines have been licensed to treat more than 180 animal disease agents. However, despite the benefits that have accompanied the development of molecular vaccines, many challenges remain. More research is required to determine the safety and efficacy of these vaccines and to develop new vaccines for the many diseases that are currently not preventable.

How are the fields of immunology and vaccinology currently developing? How can research improve the current state of these fields, and what can health professionals do to advance that research?

Animal and human health professionals from around the world addressed these and other questions at the "Advances in Immunology and Vaccine Discovery EU-US Workshop," held December 12-14 at the ARS National Animal Disease Centre in Ames, Iowa.

The USDA co-sponsored the workshop with the Office of Naval Research, the National Science Foundation, the National Institutes of Health, Iowa State University, the Molecular Vaccines Interagency Working Group, and the European Commission Directorate of Research.

Workshop attendees identified and prioritised recommendations for vaccine discovery research. These include making vaccine research a national public health priority, defining critical lists of disease agents that require new or improved vaccines, and further developing molecular vaccine technology.

During the workshop, the attendees identified some of the most serious problems facing immunology today, and developed strategies to address them. If implemented, the recommendations from this meeting will help develop new animal vaccines that could improve animal health, reduce the risk of humans contracting zoonotic diseases, improve food production efficiency and protect U.S. agriculture from foreign animal diseases.

Keeping Zoonotic Diseases in Check

They're all zoonoses—diseases that can be transmitted between humans and animals. Zoonotic diseases can create serious problems for agricultural production-—not only by harming animal and human health, but by decreasing efficiency and disrupting trade.

To help control and eradicate the most serious zoonotic diseases affecting U.S. livestock, researchers with the Agricultural Research Service (ARS) are analysing genomes, improving diagnostic platforms, studying vectors, developing vaccines and investigating the immunological responses of various animals. Below are five examples of how ARS efforts have helped reduce the impact of these diseases on the United States' agricultural industry.

Brucellosis

Brucellosis, caused by the *Brucella* bacteria, can induce fever, debilitation and miscarriages in humans, livestock and wild animals. *Brucella* can spread via physical contact or through consumption of unpasteurised milk products.

A key element of protecting livestock from brucellosis is eliminating infection in wild animals—such as bison, elk and wild swine—that share their grazing land. Although cooperative federal and state programs have nearly eliminated brucellosis in U.S. livestock, outbreaks in wild animals pose a potential threat.

One wildlife vaccination method involves firing projectile vaccines. Steven Olsen, a veterinary medical officer at the ARS National Animal Disease Centre (NADC)—part of the National Centres for Animal Health—at Ames, Iowa, collaborated with scientists at Colorado State University in Fort Collins to develop an improved vaccine pellet for bison. They found that placing the vaccine RB51 in a gel protected the vaccine's live bacteria, leading to more successful vaccinations.

NADC researchers are also evaluating novel vaccine strains—one for bison and elk and one for swine. One vaccine, developed at Virginia Tech in Blacksburg, Va., compared favourably with commercially available vaccines. Another also showed promise when administered orally or via injection.

Leptospirosis

Leptospirosis—which affects over 500,000 people globally every year—has a large host range and is one of the world's most common zoonotic diseases. It is transmitted via contact with contaminated body fluids containing spiral-shaped *Leptospira* bacteria. Mild cases resemble flu, but serious infections can lead to death.

Richard Zuerner, a NADC microbiologist, and his ARS colleagues have helped sequence the genomes of several *Leptospira* strains. Genomic studies conducted with collaborators at Monash University and the University of Queensland—both located in Australia—revealed changes in one serovar of *L. borgpetersenii* that affects cattle. Such changes could eventually limit the pathogen's ability to survive outside a mammalian host, which would reduce its effectiveness at spreading leptospirosis.

In a related study, Zuerner and his colleagues inspected tissue samples from infected animals to see if a specific bacterial protein formed when animals were infected with Leptospira. They found a protein consistent with LipL46: a "*lipoprotein*"—a membrane protein linked directly to fat molecules—identified by collaborators at UCLA. Further tests will determine whether the protein is expressed during infection or at another time.

Tuberculosis

The prevalence of bovine tuberculosis (TB) in the United States has decreased greatly since eradication efforts were first introduced in 1917. Unfortunately, the persistence of the infection in large dairy herds, imported cattle and wild animals has prevented its complete elimination.

In a biosafety level 3 facility at NADC, veterinary immunologist Ray Waters, veterinary pathologist Mitchell Palmer and molecular immunologist Tyler Thacker have evaluated the efficacy of existing vaccines and improved diagnostic assays, contributing to a significant reduction in the prevalence of TB in recent decades.

Many of their efforts target the deer—both wild and captive—that transmit it to cattle. In one project, the team collaborated with Chembio Diagnostic Systems, Inc. (Medford, N.Y.) to develop a rapid diagnostic test for the detection of TB in deer. The test uses a whole-blood sample and takes 10-15 minutes to process. The team also worked with

Prionics AG (Zurich, Switzerland) to develop improved antigens to use in TB diagnostic assays. By improving existing tools and developing new control measures, the NADC scientists have helped reduce the spread of bovine tuberculosis throughout the United States.

Rift Valley Fever

Rift Valley Fever (RVF) is a potentially fatal insect-borne disease of humans and animals, such as cattle, sheep, camels and goats. Abortions and loss of young animals are associated with RVF outbreaks. The risk of severe disease and death is much higher for livestock than for humans, but the symptoms—which include fever, aching muscles and vomiting—are unpleasant for both.

Scientists at the Arthropod-Borne Animal Diseases Research Laboratory (ABADRL) at Laramie, Wyo., are working with domestic and international collaborators to protect our nation's agricultural animals against the disease. Although RVF has not yet been introduced into the United States, it is considered a significant disease threat to U.S. livestock. The ABADRL team is cooperating with the Department of Homeland Security to assess potential vaccines for the RVF virus. In addition, the scientists are developing and evaluating diagnostic tests for RVF virus antigens.

In 2006, a team established by entomologist Kenneth J. Linthicum, director of the ARS Centre for Medical, Agricultural and Veterinary Entomology in Gainesville, Fla., produced a model that successfully predicted a Rift Valley fever outbreak in sub-Saharan Africa several months in advance. The early warning allowed organisations to advise at-risk countries to increase surveillance and insect control.

Bovine Spongiform Encephalopathy

Bovine spongiform encephalopathy (BSE, or "mad cow disease") is a deadly neurological disorder characterised by abnormally folded prions—proteins that occur naturally in mammals. In humans, the related encephalopathy, caused by the ingestion of BSE-contaminated bovine products, is known as variant Creutzfeldt-Jakob disease. In both cattle and humans, the disease causes neurological dysfunction and, eventually, death.

The United States has had only three confirmed cases of BSE. NADC scientists confirmed the first case in December 2003, and ARS scientists at the U.S. Meat Animal Research Centre in Clay Centre, Neb., traced its origin to Canada. Between June 2004 and July 2006, over 759,000 cattle have been tested for BSE, two of which tested positive. Laboratory tests showed that the manifestation of BSE in the second and third cases, which originated in the United States, differed significantly from the first. Veterinary medical officer Juergen Richt and NADC colleagues helped identify and describe the atypical cases.

In related work, Richt and his colleagues evaluated eight "prion protein knock-out" Holstein calves developed in collaboration with Hematech, Inc., a pharmaceutical research company based in Sioux Falls, S.D. These were the first cattle ever produced to lack the prion protein involved in the pathogenesis of BSE. Brain material derived from these animals was not able to support BSE-amplification when tested in an in vitro BSE amplification assay. The scientists determined that the health and growth rate of these unique animals, which will be invaluable for future BSE studies, compared to those of normal Holsteins.

Zoonotic diseases are one of several challenges facing U.S. livestock, but thanks to these and other research efforts in the ARS Animal Health National Program, our agricultural animals are among the healthiest in the world.

Stress: Compromising Animal Health

Researchers in the Livestock Behaviour Research Unit in West Lafayette, Indiana, report their studies on stress in poultry, pigs and cattle in the latest issue of *Agricultural Research.*

Whenever we feel stress—like falling off a ladder—our bodies react in predictable ways—increased heart rate, rapid and shallow breathing, and an adrenaline rush. Animals feel stress too, and it can compromise their health and ability to thrive. That, in turn, can cost producers money.

Vitamin C and beta-glucan supplements can help piglets gain weight after weaning.

Researchers in the Livestock Behaviour Research Unit in West Lafayette, Indiana, study stress in poultry, swine, and cattle.

In one study, research leader Donald C. Lay, Jr., used animal restraint and stress-inducing hormone injections of sows as stressors. He found that prenatal stress, the stress imposed on a pregnant animal, resulted in widespread effects on the offspring.

"Prenatal stress has been shown to have effects on the behaviour and physiology of many species, including monkeys, rats, guinea pigs, goats, humans, and swine," says Mr Lay. "Research in our lab has shown that prenatal stress, from restraint and stress hormone injection of sows, caused offspring to have increased plasma cortisol levels in response to stress and less ability to heal a wound when subjected to stress."

Cortisol is a glucocorticoid—a class of steroid hormones that suppress the immune system. Cortisol can also raise blood pressure and blood sugar levels.

"Prenatal stress has been shown to cause an increase in fetal cortisol, which may in turn impair immune function and increase the maximum binding capacity of glucocorticoid receptors in the central nervous system immediately after birth."

Pigs in social groups are known to form hierarchies. Sows at the bottom of the hierarchy may produce litters of prenatally stressed piglets. Mr Lay and his colleagues have shown that the effects associated with prenatal stress in swine, however, are not caused by cortisol alone. They are continuing research to identify the other factors involved.

Treating Farm Animal Stress from the Inside Out

Animal well-being can be improved and stress counteracted in farm animals by enhancing their enteric health and immunity through dietary supplements. In studies to reduce the negative health effects of a known stressor—such as animal transport and handling—animal physiologist Susan Eicher has shown that betaglucan (a yeast cell-wall product) and vitamin C supplements, fed together, can improve piglet health by enhancing the animals' growth and immune function after transport.

In Ms Eicher's studies, piglets received diets supplemented with beta-glucan alone, vitamin C alone, or both beta-glucan and vitamin C. An unsupplemented diet was fed to piglets as a control.

"Piglets receiving both vitamin C and beta-glucan had a greater weight gain after weaning," says Ms Eicher. "We also detected changes in the expression of immune-system communication molecules called 'cytokines' in intestinal and liver tissues." Other animal species may also benefit from this combination diet during stressful times, such as transport.

This ARS nutritional supplemental combination was patented in 2005 and is licensed. The marketed product is presently used by calf producers in Idaho, and they report a lower incidence of respiratory problems.

Reducing Stress—and Pain—of Birds' Beak Trimming

Beak trimming is a routine husbandry procedure used in the commercial poultry industry—particularly in broiler breeders and laying hens—to reduce injuries during confinement.

During conventional beak trimming, one-third to one-half of the beak is removed. A hot blade is normally used to cut and cauterize the beaks of chicks. But the process can be painful to the birds, so alternative methods are needed.

Biologist Heng Wei Cheng has identified a better technique—infrared laser—that can reduce pain and tissue damage.

"Infrared lasers have been widely used for noninvasive surgical procedures in human medicine and their results are reliable, predictable, and reproducible," says Mr Cheng. "Infrared lasers have recently been designed with the purpose of providing a less painful, more precise beak-trimming method compared with conventional beak trimming."

Infrared laser was compared to conventional beak trimming, and the results are promising. "Our results indicate that while there was no statistical difference in egg production or bird body weight between the two beak-trim treatments, those birds treated with the infrared method displayed superior feather condition and reduced aggression, even though they had less of the beak removed," says Mr Cheng. "The data show that infrared beak treatment may reduce the damage done by feather pecking and provides a better alternative to conventional beak trimming. Indeed, infrared trimming may provide a less invasive alternative to conventional beak trimming without compromising productivity."

These research efforts are just some of many projects of the Livestock Behaviour Research Unit that are aimed at improving existing practices and inventing new practices that enhance animal well-being and increase animal productivity.

Effects of Stockperson Behaviour on Animal Welfare & Productivity

Speaking at a recent Boehringer Animal Welfare Forum, Professor Paul Hemsworth, fDirector of the Animal Welfare Science Centre discussed human-animal interactions in livestock production. Charlotte Johnston, TheCattleSite Editor reports from the conference.

A stockpersons attitude and behaviour has a significant effect on an animals fear, welfare and productivity.

Professor Hemsworth and his colleague Professor Grahame Coleman from the Animal Welfare Science Centre focus their research on how these attitudes and behaviours affect animal welfare, and subsequently productivity.

Capacity, willingness and opportunity all affect a stockpersons work performance, said Prof Hemsworth.

Capacity is knowledge and technical skills, whilst willingness is attitudes, motivation and work ethics. Opportunity refers to the opportunity to carry out the task-which is affected by work conditions, co-workers, time available etc.

The Concept of Human-animal Relationships

Human-animal relationships can be assessed by looking at each partner's perception of the other. Frequent and intense interactions between both parties will undoubtedly develop a relationship.

So an animals perception of its relationship with humans can be studied by examining the behavioural and physiological response of the animal to humans. Similarly, the humans perception of this relationship is found by examining the behaviour and attitude of the human towards the animal.

Prof Hemsworth said that studies often focus on the animal's fear responses to humans-because of the implications on welfare.

A model of human-animal interactions in livestock industries

Handling Studies

A mixture of handling studies and field observations have been carried out, which provide significant insights into human-animal relationships, said Prof Hemsworth.

Assessing an animals relationship is done through a variety of tests.

Behavioural tests, such as response to flight distance: response to stationary human, response to moving human, response to actual handling.

Physiological tests: such as heart rates and corticosteroid (stress) responses etc.

Results have shown a substantial variation in fear responses and stockperson behaviour between farms, said Prof Hemsworth.

Human behaviour eliciting certain animal responses have been measured as positive or negative.

A negative handling behaviour, such as slaps, hits, fast movements, shouting and noise will cause an increase in fear in the animal, resulting in avoidance, stress and handling difficulties.

Positive stockperson behaviours, such as pats, strokes, talking, hand resting on the back, slow and deliberate movements will reduce the animal's level of fear of humans and result in animals which are less stressed and are easier to handle.

Prof Hemsworth's own studies, as well as more recent and past studies all show a strong correlation between negative stockperson behaviour and an increase in fear of humans.

These effects have been demonstrated in many farm animal species.

Negative Handling: Fear and Stress

Research by Breurer et al in 2003, looked at handling, fear and stress physiology in dairy cows. Dairy cows were exposed to five minutes of handling a day, for five weeks. Some animals in the study were exposed to negative handling, whilst others received positive handling. To measure the cows fear and stress, avoidance of humans (flight distance), acute cortisol response (at five minutes after human exposure) and basal free cortisol concentrations (taken in the morning) were measured.

Animals exposed to positive handling had a much shorter flight distance (humans could get much closer to the animal before it withdrew).

As well as a shorter flight time, acute cortisol responses were significantly lower, compared animals that had received negative handling.

Interestingly, the research showed that negative handling of the dairy animals resulted in higher basal free cortisol concentrations the following morning-suggesting that the animals were significantly affected by the five minutes of negative handling received the day before.

A study of cortisol concentrations in gilts by Prof Hemsworth, saw that concentrations of basal plasma cortisol were lower in gilts handled positively, than in gilts handled negatively.

Chapter 8

Negative Handling: Animal Productivity

In growing pigs, research has shown that negative and inconsistent handling increases fear responses.

One study by Prof Hemsworth looks at growth rates in pigs. His study showed that the growth rate of positively handled pigs was 455 g/ day, whereas it was only 404 g/day in pigs negatively handled. The growth rates for inconsistent pigs was 420 g/day.

In this situation, the growth rate was reduced due to the animals stress response (cortisol concentrations were elevated in inconsistent and negatively handled pigs), said Prof Hemsworth.

A similar study was carried out in laying hens, looking at the effects of negative handling (sudden and unpredictable movements in front of the pens) and positive handling (an extra two minutes spent in front of the cages, and slow deliberate movements).

Hen time at the front of the cage was measured, with less time at the front of cage took as avoidance of human contact. Stress responses and egg production were also measured. The results show that positive handling of birds means that the hens were keen to have increased human contact (less fearful), spending more time at the front of the cage.

The corticosterone stress levels were much higher in hens handled negatively, than in positively handled hens.

Subsequently egg production in the hens was eight per cent higher in hens that had a positive human-animal relationship.

The number of studies across species with strong correlations between stress and negative handling, leaves no doubt that negative handling evokes stress, affecting animal welfare and production, said Prof Hemsworth.

Negative Handling: Animal Health

As mentioned above, studies have shown that negative handling affects an animals fear of humans, leading to stress, which consequently affects health.

One study shows that socialised (used to positive human contact, so less fear) birds had higher feed conversion efficiency. In this same study, birds that were less socialised (more fear of humans) had higher lesions and deaths, as well as overall poorer health.

Prof Hemsworth says this is due to the response of immune system, suppressing antibodies when an animal is stressed, leading to poor health.

A different study, carried out on veal calves, looked at average daily gain and mortality. Fast movements by stockpersons were negatively associated with daily liveweight gain. As well as this, negative behaviour was seen to increase mortality, although unit size was a large variable in this study.

Longer flight distances in dairy cattle, also have a positive correlation with lameness in dairy cattle. In a study of 36 dairy heifers, 48 per cent of heifers with a flight distance of 4.8m (to humans) were lame, and on average milk yields were 1.3 kg/day less, than those with a shorter flight distance.

To compare, of cows with a flight distance of 2.81m (those that were less fearful), only six per cent showed signs of lameness.

On pasture based systems, Prof Hemsworth said that lameness in dairy cows was affected by two significant factors-the condition of farm tracks and farmers' patience in the dairy, ie. their behaviour towards cows.

What is an attitude, asks Prof Hemsworth. It is something that affects our behaviour and although they are stable and resistant, attitudes are learnt.

They are shaped through direct and indirect experiences, therefore throughout one's lifespan, attitudes can be changed.

Professor Hemsworth says to change stockperson behaviour, it is important to target attitudes as well.

Cognitive-behavioural Training

Evidence from studies carried out by Prof Hemsworth and colleagues suggests that stockperson training can improve animal productivity and welfare.

To change the behaviour of stockpeople towards farm animals ultimately requires:

- targeting the beliefs that underlie the behaviour,
- targeting the behaviour in question, and
- then maintaining these changed beliefs and behaviours.

One study looked at the benefits of cognitive-behavioural training on dairy units. The key variables measured were stockperson attitudes, stockperson behaviours, fear of humans and animal productivity.

The study demonstrated that training significantly improved stockperson attitudes. Training also halved stockperson negative behaviour towards cattle. Whilst the fear responses of cows didn't change much, the changes were small but significant, said Prof Hemsworth. Flight distance did not decrease a lot, but milk cortisol levels did often decline.

A second study looked at the effects of training on cow productivity at 94 dairy farms. After training, which targeted stockperson attitudes and behaviour, milk yield per cow increased, as did the protein and fat content of the milk produced.

Stockperson Selection

Some studies, by the Animal Welfare Science Centre, have looked at how the selection of a stockperson can improve animal welfare.

Measuring stockperson characteristics prior to employment, may give employers an idea of stockperson attitudes and consequently behaviour towards animals.

Concluding, Prof Hemsworth said that the role of a stockperson in animal welfare and productivity should not be underestimated. The studies in this article are just a few of the many that have been carried out. The outcomes highlight how important the role of the stockperson is in developing positive human animal relationships, and consequently improving animal welfare and productivity.

Natural Alternative to Antibiotics in Animal Feed

Binding molecules from seaweed extracts within the molecular layers of natural clays makes the clay ten times more efficient at adsorbing the harmful fungal toxins which are commonly found in animal feed. The resulting new hybrid product has a huge potential market worldwide as a completely natural, effective alternative to the formerly-used antibiotics, which are now prohibited from this use in the European Union.

EUREKA project E! 3025 Monlisa has developed a new, completely natural alternative to using antibiotics in animal feed. Formerly used as growth promoters and to prevent the damaging effects of the fungal toxins which are often present in feed, antibiotics have been prohibited for use in animal feed in the EU since 2006 – creating a need for a new, effective antimycotoxic agent. The already-known capacity of clay minerals to adsorb these mycotoxins has been increased ten times over in this project by the incorporation of molecules of extracts from algae (seaweed) onto the clay. The resulting activated clay is added to animal feed, where it is highly efficient at adsorbing the mycotoxin molecules.

Mycotoxins – which have, over the years, become one of the major concerns of animal feed producers – are the chemical products of fungal moulds which are often present in cereal grains and forage crops. They are especially prevalent in warm and humid regions like Asia and South America, where the climate conditions favour fungal growth. Mycotoxins cause a range of problems to farm animals, including reducing their feed intake and therefore reducing their growth. Consuming mycotoxins can also make animals more susceptible to disease and lead to damaged liver and kidneys. Human health is affected by consumption of animal products like meat, milk and eggs which are contaminated with mycotoxins.

For many years, a range of antibiotics have been applied in low doses to animal feed, to control the production of mycotoxins and to act as growth promoters. But as part of its policy to reduce the threat of developing microbial resistance to antibiotics, the use of antibiotics in animal feed was banned in the EU from 1 January 2006. This policy meant that there was an urgent need for some other way to control the mycotoxins in animal feed.

Multiple Applications

French company Olmix was aware that some naturally occurring clay minerals, particularly montmorillonite, were able to adsorb organic molecules including these toxic substances onto their surface. The clays are formed of layers of about one nanometre. Within the Monalisa project, French company Olmix employed the process known as intercalation, to include molecules of seaweed extracts between the clay layers; making the new product Amadeite®. This process separates the layers (delamination) and increases the interlayer space; and as a result the clay is able to adsorb up to ten times the amount of mycotoxins compared to pure clay.

Dr Anca Laza-Knoerr says: "Our idea was to introduce a natural product into the clay, rather than the synthetic polymers that had already been used to make activated clays."

The process, which involves suspension of the clay and seaweed extract in water, followed by removal of the remaining algal extract, centrifugation and drying, now holds two worldwide patents. It is the development of this process that is the main technological innovation. As well as applications in the field of animal feed, the clay-algal extract combination has potential uses in the purification of water from waste effluents, heavy metals or radioactive pollution.

Olmix worked on the preparation of the seaweed for extraction in partnership with other specialised laboratories: the European Research Centre for Algae (CEVA) and the Laboratoire de Matériaux à Porosité Contrôlée (LMPC, Mulhouse). The seaweed is readily and cheaply available on beaches but it has to be carefully washed before extraction so that residual sand does not damage the extraction machinery. Use of the algae for this purpose has the secondary benefit that it is so plentiful in some regions that it is considered an environmental pollutant.

Successful Products from Basic Research

Further development of the application of Amadeite® in animal feed was made by the Spanish partner in the Monalisa project, Adiveter, which has specialist knowledge of the microbiological monitoring of feeds and raw materials. As a result, since the end of the project Olmix has been able to market two products for use in animal feed. The first, called M Feed, is a growth promoter which aids the digestive process and helps to maintain the balance of the gut microflora. The economic yield of the animals is increased by enhanced digestion and growth. The second product, MTx+ adsorbs harmful mycotoxins from the feed and its use has been shown to increase livestock productivity. Both products are already being marketed in many countries throughout Europe and in Russia, the US and Japan, with estimated worldwide sales of €12 million in 2009.

Aurélie Garel, also from Olmix, said: "The activated clay Amadeite is an innovative, natural additive, and really important for agriculture and many other industrial applications."

Developing the new activated clay product Amadeite was only possible through the support of EUREKA, which helped to locate and bring together partner organisations with the right expertise and facilities. Collaboration between the partner organisations was excellent. The impact of the project is that it allowed the development of a highly effective range of products, to take the place of the antibiotics whose widespread use was threatening to increase microbial resistance.

Economic Impacts of Foreign Animal Disease

This report by the USDA Economic Research Service presents a modelling framework in which epidemiological model results are integrated with an economic model of the U.S. agricultural sector to enable estimation of the economic impacts of outbreaks of foreign-source livestock diseases. It was produced by Philip L. Paarlberg, Ann Hillberg Seitzinger, John G. Lee and Kenneth H. Mathews, Jr.

Summary

This study uses a modelling framework to estimate the nature of economic impacts of outbreaks of foreign-source livestock diseases. The model is more comprehensive than previous work because (1) it has components for modelling both economic effects and disease-spread effects from an outbreak, for which the results can be integrated; (2) it assesses the effects of a disease outbreak on major agricultural sectors—livestock and crops—along vertical market chains, from production to consumption; and (3) it projects the impacts of the disease outbreak over 20 calendar quarters, rather than for just 1 year.

What is the Issue?

As more is learned about the impacts of foreign animal disease outbreaks, questions arise regarding the efficiency of existing animal disease-impact models for capturing the array of effects across many economic sectors and over time. Previous models lacked adequate treatment of either the economic components or the epidemiological components, and, in some cases, both. Further, there is a need to address the ways that alternative control strategies affect the economic interests of the numerous agricultural sectors, both on and off the farm.

What are the Major Findings?

While the framework can be applied to many livestock diseases, this study demonstrates the model with a hypothetical outbreak of foot-and-mouth disease (FMD). The outbreak is assumed to occur in small hog operations in the U.S. Midwest, a result of using contaminated garbage as feed. Various disease-control strategies are entered into the model. The economic effects from each control strategy are based on 50 iterations of the disease-outbreak epidemiological model, which randomly assigns different herd sizes, spatial distribution, and other variables for each iteration. The model produced the following key results:

- Epidemiological model results show that relatively few animals need to be destroyed because of the disease.
- Economic model results show large monetary losses for beef, beef cattle, hogs, and pork sectors, mainly caused by the loss of exports under a given set of foreign sanitary and phytosanitary policies. Other agricultural sectors experience small losses or, in some cases, small gains.
- Swine and pork sectors recover shortly after export restrictions end, while effects on beef and cattle sectors last longer due to the longer cattle production cycle.
- Disease control strategies that reduce the duration of the outbreak are the most effective choices for reducing the economic toll. The model found that three strategies reduce the duration to less than one quarter. In order of least to most effective, based on the mean number of days to end the outbreak, for the hypothetical outbreak these are:
    - o Destruction of only those herds within a radius of 1 km that have had direct contact with infected herds: Outbreaks average 56.48 days.
    - o Direct-and-indirect-contact slaughter, which destroys direct contact herds plus those herds indirectly exposed to an infected herd through movement of people, vehicles, or other possible sources of infection: Outbreaks average 54.99 days.
    - o Destruction of all herds within a 1 km radius of the initial outbreak: Outbreaks average 36.8 days.
- Export embargoes increase domestic meat supplies, and domestic consumers benefit from lower prices during the quarters in which exports are embargoed.
- Model results, extended to 16 quarters, show that for this hypothetical outbreak:
    - o After 7 quarters, production of all commodities increases to the point where both domestic consumption and trade return to predisease levels.

- o Total trade losses, plus other disease-related costs to capital and management, amount to between $2,773 million and $4,062 million, compared with a disease-free baseline period (2001-2004).

How was the Study Conducted?

The framework has two components: (1) The North American Animal Disease-spread Model (NAADSM), developed by the U.S. Department of Agriculture's Animal and Plant Health Inspection Service, which enables estimates of epidemiological damages (supply shocks) from varying diseasespread and control scenarios. These estimates can then be integrated with (2) an economic model, developed by Paarlberg, Seitzinger, and Lee, that assesses effects of supply shocks from the epidemiological model, along with demand and trade shocks, projected over the simulation period.

To illustrate the modelling framework, a hypothetical outbreak of FMD arising from feeding garbage in four small farrow-to-finish operations is examined under three alternative control strategies and three levels of disease intensity. The control strategies are (1) destruction of direct-contact herds, (2) destruction of direct-contact and indirect-contact herds, and (3) destruction of all animals within a 1-km ring. Disease intensity is examined at low, medium, and high levels. Each disease control scenario was simulated 50 times, with the epidemiological model determining effects of an outbreak.

Animal losses and duration of the FMD outbreak are sensitive to the conditions assumed for the outbreak, i.e., that it started on small pig farms and was confined to them. Alternative scenarios could result in higher costs than reported in this analysis. Future work will evaluate the robustness of these results.

Variation in Costs for Animal Disease Prevention

A new report *Cost of National Prevention Systems for Animal Diseases and Zoonoses in Developing and Transition Countries* commissioned by the World Organisation for Animal Health (OIE) has been published recently. The main conclusions are summarised by Jackie Linden for TheCattleSite. These include that there is a strong relationship between current spending per animal unit and GDP, although this is unrelated to the level of spending required.

The OIE commissioned Civic Consulting to conduct a study on the cost of National Prevention Systems (NPS) for animal diseases and zoonoses in developing and transition countries.

The final report explains that the aims of the study were two-fold:

1. to estimate the 'peace time' costs of Veterinary Services allowing early detection and rapid response to emerging and re-emerging diseases in different regions, economies, animal health systems and eco-systems, and
2. to develop economic indicators within the OIE-PVS Tool for the Evaluation of Performance of Veterinary Services (OIE-PVS Tool).

The study was based on the results of in-depth research in nine OIE member countries (Costa Rica, Kyrgyzstan, Mongolia, Morocco, Romania, Turkey, Uganda, Uruguay, Viet Nam) and an extensive analysis of possible economic indicators.

The study team, led by Dr Frank Alleweldt (project director) and Professor Martin Upton (lead author of the economic analysis), drew 11 main conclusions.

NPS Expenditure is Related to Livestock Population

One leading conclusion in the report is that substantial differences in the public expenditure for the National Prevention System for Animal Diseases and Zoonoses exist between case study countries, reaching from 10 million international dollars to 167 million international dollars. The average expenditure on the National Prevention System was 48.6 million international dollars in the baseline year, 2007.

Variations in expenditures between case study countries are clearly associated with differences in livestock population. Operational costs of the National Prevention System, when expressed on a per Veterinary Livestock Units (VLU) basis, therefore give a comparative measure of the level of service provision in relation to the quantitative requirements.

NPS Expenditure is Correlated with GDP

In the case study countries, there is a close relationship between Gross Domestic Product (GDP) and the total public expenditures for the National Prevention System. Differences in GDP explain to a large degree the variation in NPS expenditures.

NPS expenditure appears to be mainly dependent on the country's ability to pay, rather than on the veterinary requirements. This may lead to a significant under-funding of the NPS, most notably in low-income countries. In these cases, veterinary services require a higher priority in the national budget allocation, and/or sustained external support to be able to effectively address global animal health challenges.

Strong Relationship between Spending per Animal Unit and Incomes

Differences in NPS expenditures between countries on a per VLU basis are, at least partly, explained by differences in per capita incomes, according to the report.

While the overall average NPS cost per VLU for the seven countries amounts to 5.66 international dollars, the average for the three low-income countries – Uganda, Kyrgyzstan and Viet Nam – is only 3.82 international dollars. The average for the two lower-middle-income countries – Mongolia and Morocco – is 5.28 international dollars, while that for the upper-middle-income countries – Costa Rica and Turkey – is 8.79 international dollars.

Total Cost Per Animal Unit is not Affected by the Level of Centralisation

Sub-national expenditures tend to increase relative to the centralised expenditures with increasing size of the national territory. Operating expenditures associated with the National Prevention System are incurred either centrally, in or near the main centre of government, or dispersed more widely in provincial, regional or district locations.

A high central expenditure in Costa Rica is clearly associated with a centralised structure in a relatively small country, whereas Turkey, Morocco and Vietnam, three of the largest countries in area, spent about three-quarters of the total NPS operating expenditure at the sub-national level.

Provided that both central and regional elements are included, the average total cost per VLU may be unaffected by the extent of decentralised expenditure, say the report's authors.

No Explanation Found for Differences in Spending Patterns

Spending patterns for different categories of expenditures varied between the case study countries, however, this provides little explanation for differences in overall NPS expenditures. Levels of staff costs and expenditures such as travel costs appear to be directly related to levels of per capita income of case study countries.

Considerable differences in spending that depend on other factors are related to three categories:

- fees for private veterinarians conducting public service mission (up to 0.96 international dollar/VLU)
- expenditures for vaccines (up to 1.57 international dollar/VLU), and
- compensation of livestock holders (up to 0.74 international dollar/VLU).

In some other countries, spending for these items is zero or close to zero.

Public NPS Expenditure is not Related to the Strength of the Private Sector

There is no evidence that a stronger private veterinary sector reduces public NPS expenditures in the case study countries. The relative strength of the private veterinary sector, expressed as the ratio of public to private veterinarians, appears to be related to the income level of the country.

In the case study countries, both NPS expenditures and the relative importance of the private veterinary sector increase with a higher GNI per capita.

GDP Does not Correlate with NPS Requirement

The strong linear correlation between GDP and NPS expenditures for the case study countries can be used to estimate current National Prevention System expenditure. However, this approach provides a rough estimation of the likely current level of funding of the NPS only, and does not in any case determine the optimal level of NPS expenditures in a given country.

The only reliable and accurate method of obtaining data on NPS expenditures in other countries currently available is by means of direct measurement, using the methodology developed for this study.

System to Quantify Results is Needed

The report's authors suggest that a quantitative expression of OIE-PVS Evaluation (OIE-PVS Tool for the Evaluation of Performance of Veterinary Services) results would be helpful for assessing the degree of compliance with OIE International Standards on Quality of Veterinary Services in a systemic perspective.

In future refinements of the PVS Tool, the introduction of a more quantitative approach could be considered. Also, due to the cross-cutting character of several of the critical competencies used for the

PVS Tool, it is currently difficult to correlate the costs for key NPS elements (e.g. veterinary diagnostic laboratories) to the results of a sub-set of PVS critical competencies related to this NPS element.

It could therefore also be considered to refine and group critical competencies to allow a more direct correlation of PVS results and costs for key elements of the NPS.

Governments to Keep a Record of PVS staff

OIE member countries should collect data on staff numbers of the public Veterinary Services across all levels of government.

Although collection of such data would require additional efforts by member governments, this would hugely improve the basis for any future economic assessment of the National Prevention System, as staff costs account for up to three-quarters of NPS operating expenditures in the case study countries. This could be encouraged by revising the reporting format for the annual OIE World Animal Health Report.

A possible reporting format, suggested in this study, would differentiate between public and private veterinary personnel, differentiate the categories of veterinary personnel paid from the public budget and differentiate the type of activity of the personnel.

Standards should be Established for Future Comparisons

A 'gold standard' or quality benchmark figures are needed from the OIE for comparison of NPS expenditures between countries, but assessments may be more effective if focused on key elements rather than on the total NPS expenditure at national level.

The authors says that the results of their study suggest a gradual approach to derive benchmark values that provide guidance to countries for allocating their NPS expenditures effectively and efficiently, focusing on key elements of the National Prevention System (such as cost of surveillance, border inspection, diagnostic laboratory facilities).

Benchmarking of Costs would Aid Budgeting

Finally, the authors recommend that consideration should be given to the development of a database of benchmark cost data concerning specific components of NPS expenditures. The necessary data could be obtained during the PVS Evaluation or PVS Gap Analysis visit or, alternatively, through a visit of a specialist expert team.

Benchmark cost data concerning key elements of the NPS would create a better basis for the design and budgeting of desired improvements in the NPS provisions in developing and transition countries, creating both a better basis for the budgeting process of specific countries and more transparency for donors.

Animal Cloning and Implications for the Food Chain

This report examines the potential issues involved with cloning animals for commercial industry, prepared for COI, on behalf of their client, The Food Standards Agency.

Executive Summary

Background

Animal cloning is an emerging technology in the EU (although already more established in the US), and there is potential that, if its use becomes economically viable, food derived from cloned animals will enter the food chain across the world.

It is thought that this topic is likely to encounter a significant amount of consumer interest as the technology develops. For this reason, the Food Standards Agency commissioned research to explore initial public perceptions of animal cloning and to identify what the key issues and areas of concern/uncertainty are, particularly in relation to food.

Research Objectives

The overall aims of the research were to inform the development of the Agency's communication around this issue, to ensure that the consumer is fully informed of all aspects of the technology and to ensure that all areas of potential public concern are addressed when the acceptability of cloned animals for food production is being assessed in the EU and therefore becomes an issue more visible to the general public.

The research objectives addressed the following key areas:

1. Perceptions of current farming practices including breeding practices and views on cloning as an assisted reproductive technology
2. Levels of knowledge and perceived benefits of animal cloning
3. Animal welfare issues and other ethical concerns
4. Safety concerns in relation to food derived from clones and their offspring
5. Views on the need for, and nature of, regulation of animal cloning

6. Views on labelling of foodstuffs linked to cloned animals
7. Views on the role of the FSA in relation to this new technology.

Research Method

Given the complex nature of the topic and the evidence from previous research that public awareness and understanding of the issues are limited, a deliberative approach was adopted based on reconvened workshops, with participants taking part in two three hour sessions as well as carrying out their own background reading and research. The first workshop focused on current livestock breeding methods, an explanation of how clones are produced, how this technique can be applied to animal livestock breeding and the implications of this for the food chain. The second workshop focused on participants' views on buying and eating food derived from clones and their offspring as well as the steps they thought should be taken if such food went on sale in the UK.

Four sets of workshops were conducted, one in each of England, Scotland, Wales and Northern Ireland.

Key Findings

Current Animal Livestock Breeding

- It was accepted that livestock breeders actively manage the process in order to ensure they breed from their 'best' animals. With the exception of artificial insemination, most people had not heard of the various forms of assisted reproductive technologies currently in use
- In this context, most participants felt animal cloning represents a quantum leap from 'giving mother nature a helping hand' to 'interfering with mother nature'.

Understanding of Cloning and Perceived Benefits

- Initial levels of knowledge about, and understanding of, cloning varied widely.
- Participants struggled to identify any convincing benefits of the technique. They felt the only 'winners' were likely to be biotech companies, livestock breeders, farmers or food retailers and they were concerned that the main motive for introducing animal cloning was a pecuniary one. They questioned whether consumers would derive any tangible benefits.

Animal Welfare and Other Ethical Issues

- As participants learned about the current low efficiency rates of the cloning method they became increasingly concerned about the implications for animal welfare. This became a significant factor behind their reluctance to accept food derived from clones and their offspring.
- The research highlighted a number of other concerns that the public are likely to voice in relation to the use of animal cloning for food production. These included concerns about where the technology might lead (in particular, to human cloning) and whether mankind has the moral right to pursue such a course.
- Underpinning many of their concerns was a lack of trust in the various players involved including biotech companies, scientists, livestock breeders, farmers, government, food manufacturers and retailers.
- If the FSA, or any other body, wishes to be a credible and reliable source of independent advice in this area, it is essential that it is seen to transcend the needs and aspirations of these different players.

Safety Concerns in Relation to Food Derived from Clones

- Opinions were shaped by previous events especially in relation to BSE/vCJD and GM food.
- Many participants were concerned that cloning could result in food that was unsafe for human consumption. This was partly a function of the perceived high incidence of miscarriages and deformed and short-lived offspring resulting from the process. It was also because of a fear that the process of cloning might somehow create new diseases or affect the food in some way that will be harmful to humans.
- There were also concerns that cloning might impact on food quality, consistency, uniformity and price.
- There is a major mismatch between the methods used by regulatory authorities to assess food safety and the public's perception of what is needed. Participants wanted to see methods for assessing food safety that were analogous to the approach used in clinical drugs trials.
- If the efficiency of cloning can be greatly improved, this will lessen the idea that the resulting offspring may pose food

safety concerns. However, unless the mismatch in perceptions about the required method of assessing food safety can be addressed, the public are likely to harbour major concerns that such food is unsafe to eat.

The Need for Regulation of Animal Cloning

- If food derived from clones and their offspring were to go on sale in the UK, the research has provided a clear steer in terms of the steps that would help to increase consumer confidence. Irrespective of how participants felt about buying and eating such food, there was a high level of agreement about how it should be introduced and regulated.

This included:

- o regulations that address the entire process from animal breeding and welfare to food production and human health, including the import and export of clones, their offspring and semen/embryos, and food derived from such
- o some form of licensing not only of the process of cloning animals but also covering how such animals enter the food chain
- o an agreed set of standards and procedures coupled with proactive monitoring and enforcement
- o traceability of clones and their offspring.

- Informing and educating the public about current regulations may help increase consumer confidence when coupled with (possibly) new controls on who can clone, how they do it and how such animals end up in the food chain.

Views on Labelling

- There was a call for all food derived from cloned animals and their offspring to be clearly labelled-not just from a food safety perspective but to enable consumers to make an informed choice. The greatest challenge lies in working out how far removed an animal needs to be from a cloned ancestor before it is considered 'normal'.

Role of the Food Standards Agency

- The FSA – possibly in partnership with other bodies-was seen by most as having a key role to play in the debate about food derived from clones and their offspring both in terms of setting and policing the rules as well as informing and educating the public.

- Whatever its role, it is crucial that it is perceived to be independent and trustworthy.

Gender Differences

- There was evidence of a clear gender divide. Men often took a more rational approach, were somewhat less concerned about, and more willing to consider buying and eating, food derived from clones and their offspring. Women seemed to engage at a more emotional level, often as mothers/grandmothers, and were more worried about animal welfare and food safety. As a result, they were more likely to reject the idea of buying/ eating such food. Given the fact that women tend to be the main food shoppers in many households, their views on such food are likely to have the greatest impact on any future uptake.

Conclusions

The key areas of concern that participants expressed are summarised below:

Based on this research, if the general public are to accept the idea of buying and eating food derived from clones and their offspring, each of these concerns would need to be addressed.

The Use of Animals in Biomedical Research: Improving Human and Animal Health

Animals used in biomedical research help us:

- understand how our bodies work
- find cures and treatments for diseases
- test new drugs for safety
- evaluate medical procedures before they are used on people.

Why Do We have to Use Animals in Research?

Although animals appear to be very different from us, their bodies work in many of the same ways ours do. Researchers who study animals discover information that can't be learned from other sources. Biomedical research saves lives. Research using animals improves the lives of millions of people each year by giving doctors clues to prevent, treat, and cure illnesses like cancer, diabetes, and AIDS. New drugs and treatments for diseases are tested on animals to make sure they are safe for people to use.

What Kinds of Animals are Used in Research?

Laboratory mice are used more often in research every year than any other animal species. Mice, and other rodents such as rats and hamsters, make up over 90% of the animals used in biomedical research. In addition to having bodies that work similar to humans and other animals, rodents are small in size, easy to handle, relatively inexpensive to buy and keep, and produce many offspring in a short period of time.

However, rodents may not always be the best animal model to use in certain experiments. In these cases, dogs, cats, rabbits, sheep, pigs, fish, frogs, birds, nonhuman primates, or other kinds of animals may be used. All of these animals together make up less than 10% of the animals used in research.

Why Can't We Use other Methods?

We use other methods whenever we can. Computer models and cell tissue studies are used in addition to animal research to discover new ways of solving complex problems. By studying cells in test tubes, scientists can learn much about how our bodies work, react to disease, and respond to treatment. Computer simulations also aid researchers. But cells and computer models simply cannot mimic the complexities of our bodies. And that's where animals come in.

Because of biomedical research we have:

- heart by-pass and other life-saving surgeries
- organ transplantation
- vaccines to prevent childhood diseases
- many other treatments and cures for diseases.

Together for Life

In the last century, most medical discoveries were possible because of animal research. To build on the great progress we've made in understanding and treating diseases, we need to continue these studies.

Cures for diseases such as cancer, AIDS, Alzheimer's disease, diabetes, cystic fibrosis, and muscular dystrophy are in reach, thanks to the animals used in research. Only through the humane use of animals in research can we hope to continue to improve the lives of both animals and humans. We all owe them a debt of gratitude for the part they play in saving the lives of millions of people around the world.

The Judicious Use of Antimicrobials for Animal Producers

To achieve that goal, producers should be committed to the practice of disease prevention through the use of vaccines, parasite control, stress reduction, environmental management and proper nutritional management. Responsible and timely management practices can reduce the incidence of disease and therefore reduce the need for antimicrobials; however, antimicrobials remain a necessary tool to manage infectious disease in beef herds.

Prudent use of antimicrobials is important to reduce livestock pain and suffering as well as minimise losses due to disease. Furthermore responsible antimicrobial use will help minimise antimicrobial resistance in bacteria, which can impact animal health in your operation and the safety of food you produce.

Like other species, bacteria find ways to survive. Whenever bacteria are exposed to antimicrobials, some survive by developing resistance. Resistance depends upon the type and amount of antimicrobial used, the number of animals treated, and the length of treatment. Therefore, it is vital to use antimicrobials appropriately and judiciously in animals under your care.

Antimicrobial resistance concerns are shared by producers, veterinarians, governmental agencies, the public health community and consumers. Of particular concern is the risk of developing antimicrobial resistant bacteria in animals and the potential for subsequent human exposure. The antimicrobial resistant bacteria can, for example, be consumed by humans along with the meat product. Producers must be committed to appropriate and judicious antibiotic use in order to (1) minimise the risk of antibiotic resistant bacteria in animals, (2) maintain the long-term effectiveness of antimicrobials for humans and livestock, and (3) protect future antimicrobial availability.

Judicious Antimicrobial Use Guidelines

Producers do not stand alone in addressing this issue. Various veterinary groups have developed and adopted judicious antimicrobial use guidelines. These guidelines provide a road map for proper antimicrobial therapeutic use in livestock.

Prevent Disease

- Prevent disease through management by emphasizing animal husbandry, biosecurity, and health maintenance. Antibiotic use cannot replace sound management practices.

- Appropriate and timely management practices include:
  - o Vaccinations
  - o Parasite control
  - o Stress reduction
  - o Nutritional management
  - o Environmental management.

Diagnose Sick Animals

- Sick animals indicate a breakdown in preventative practices.
  - o Diagnose problems early and accurately.
  - o Many diseases have similar symptoms/signs.
  - o Not all diseases are treatable with antimicrobials.
  - o Use your veterinarian and a laboratory to help diagnose the problem.

Select Appropriate Antibiotics

- Use veterinary advice and laboratory results to help select appropriate antibiotics or treatment alternatives.
- Select and use antimicrobials carefully and only when justified.
- Develop written treatment protocols in collaboration with your veterinarian.
- Use the proper dose, given by the proper route for the proper length of time.
- Treatment programs should reflect best use principles.
- Treat the fewest number of animals possible.
- Withhold treated animals or animal products properly.
- Antimicrobial use, other than according to the label and, outside of a valid veterinarian-client patient-relationship (VCPR), is a violation of federal law.

Keep Records

- Record animal or group identification, drug used, date treated, dosage used, route and location for administration, and who administered the product.
- Review records before marketing to ensure proper meat withdrawal.
- Keep and review records.
- "You cannot manage what you do not measure."

How should this Work on Your Operation?

Have a VCPR

One of the basic principles of proper antibiotic usage is having a working relationship with your veterinarian, commonly called a VCPR. This means your veterinarian knows your operation, your management, your livestock, and is involved in diagnosis and treatment decisions.

Your veterinarian must be available for follow-up in case of adverse reactions or treatment failure. This also means that you are willing to follow his/her instructions for antibiotic usage. A VCPR is not just having someone write a prescription, sell you drugs, or make them available to you.

The law requires a valid VCPR if an antibiotic is administered in any manner other than expressly stated on the label or the antibiotic is a prescription product. It is a good idea to get your veterinarian's advice on the use of any drug in your operation.

A Valid Veterinarian-client-patient Relationship is One in Which

A veterinarian has assumed the responsibility for making medical judgments regarding the health of (an) animal(s) and the need for medical treatment, and the client (the owner of the animal or animals or other caretaker) has agreed to follow the instructions of the veterinarian; (2) There is sufficient knowledge of the animal(s) by the veterinarian to initiate at least a general or preliminary diagnosis of the medical condition of the animal(s); and (3) The practicing veterinarian is readily available for follow-up in case of adverse reactions or failure of the regimen of therapy. Such a relationship can exist only when the veterinarian has recently seen and is personally acquainted with the keeping and care of the animal(s) by virtue of examination of the animal(s), and/or by medically appropriate and timely visits to the premises where the animal(s) are kept.

Establish Written Protocols

A written protocol serves as a guide for on-farm diagnosis and treatment decisions. A complete protocol should include signs of the disease and detailed directions for treatment, including meat withdrawal times. You should establish written protocols for any antimicrobial use on your operation. These protocols must include your veterinarian's input if prescription drugs are used or if drugs are used other than according to the label (extralabel use).

Extralabel Drug Use (ELDU)

Extralabel use means actual use or intended use of a drug in an animal in a manner that is not in accordance with the approved labelling. This includes, but is not limited to, use in species not listed in the labelling, use for indications (disease or other conditions) not listed in the labelling, use at dosage levels, frequencies, or routes of administration other than those stated in the labelling, and deviation from the labelled withdrawal time based on these different uses.

Understand What Constitutes Extralabel Drug Use (ELDU)

Drugs are approved by the FDA for treatment of specific diseases or conditions in a specific species or class of animal, at specific dose(s), route(s), duration(s), and frequency(s) of administration with a corresponding slaughter withdrawal time. Any use that deviates from the label instructions constitutes extralabel drug use and requires a valid VCPR.

An example of extralabel drug use is buying procaine penicillin G at a farm store and using it in cattle at a dose higher than specified on the label. The label dosage is 1 cc(ml) per 100 lb of body weight, but it is commonly used at higher dosages and/or given under the skin rather than in the muscle.

These are extralabel uses, and it is important to understand that non-prescription drugs require a valid VCPR and appropriate labelling for extralabel use. Because approved withdrawal times are based on label directions, any other use may result in residues in violation of federal law.

Prohibited Extralabel Uses

The following drugs are prohibited for extralabel use in food-producing animals (current as of May 2002)

a. Chloramphenicol;

b. Clenbuterol;

c. Diethylstilbestrol (DES);

d. Dimetridazole;

e. Ipronidazole;

f. Other nitroimidazoles;

g. Furazolidone;

h. Nitrofurazone;

i. Sulfonamide drugs in lactating dairy cattle (except approved use of sulfadimethoxine, sulfabromomethazine and sulfaethoxypyridazine);

j. Fluoroquinolones; and

k. Glycopeptides.

An example of an illegal extralabel drug usage would be the administration of fluoroquinolones (e.g. enrofloxacin) to treat calf diarrhea.

It is illegal to use any feed additive drug in an extralabel manner in beef cattle.

Train People Who Treat Livestock on Your Operation

People responsible for treating livestock must be properly trained to recognise common signs of disease as well as proper drug use and record keeping. Periodic and timely review of written protocols and treatment records with your veterinarian is the most effective method for ensuring judicious antibiotic use.

Other sources of information regarding proper use of antibiotics include extension specialists, producer associations and pharmaceutical technical service representatives. However, recommendations for extralabel usage can only be obtained from your veterinarian.

Foot and Mouth Disease: Novel Technologies Improve Detection and Control

Scientists at the USDA Agricultural Research Service (ARS) are using infrared technology to identify cattle infected with foot and mouth disease (FMD) virus. The same group has developed the world's first molecular-based FMD vaccine, which has been effective in pigs, writes Laura McGinnis, ARS staff.

Infrared thermography (IRT) cameras can see what human eyes cannot: heat. That is why scientists at the ARS Plum Island Animal Disease Centre (PIADC) at Orient Point, New York, are using the technology to identify cattle that may have been infected with foot-and-mouth disease (FMD).

"This IRT technology has been used for years and has applications for a variety of fields, from astronomy to law enforcement to the military," says PIADC research leader, Luis Rodriguez. "This is the first scientific report of IRT as a tool for early detection of FMD-infected animals."

Chemist Marvin Grubman and visiting scientist Fayna Diaz-San Segundo examine a plate used in a test to determine the correct amount of a new foot-and-mouth disease vaccine to administer to cattle.

The United States has not had an outbreak of FMD since 1929 but there is no way to guarantee that this very contagious disease is gone forever – as the United Kingdom learned in 2001, when an outbreak of FMD ended a 34-year disease-free streak. The disease spreads rapidly and wreaks havoc on trade and transportation, so being prepared for an outbreak is a priority for the US government.

An essential component of containment and eradication is the ability to quickly assess the scope of an outbreak.

"It's a huge endeavour to examine the animals one by one. Even on a small farm it's a big task," says Dr Rodriguez. He and his colleagues evaluated a new method for rapidly and accurately detecting animals at risk of infection. Their method, which uses IRT cameras to identify potentially infected animals quickly, is not intended to be a diagnostic test. Rather, it enables scientists to concentrate their resources by quickly isolating animals that require further testing with a disease-specific method.

IRT cameras can identify at-risk cattle 48 hours before they begin to show any clinical symptoms. In the event of an outbreak, this technology could facilitate rapid containment of the disease.

Spotting Hot Hooves

Infrared image of a cow not infected with foot-and-mouth disease virus (above). Note that the hooves are not red. Red colour in the hooves would indicate heat.

Infrared image of a cow infected with foot-and-mouth-disease virus. Note that the hooves are red. Red colour in the hooves indicates heat.

How does it work? Objects of all temperatures above absolute zero (about minus 460°F) emit infrared radiation. The hotter the object, the higher the emissions, and IRT cameras make those emissions visible.

Foot temperatures rise in cattle infected with the FMD virus, resulting in a visible difference in IRT photographs. This phenomenon was observed by Craig Packer, a wildlife biologist at the University of Minnesota. While tracking migratory animal populations in Africa for an unrelated study, Dr Packer used an infrared camera to take photographs of wild mammals and observed that some impala had very hot heads and feet. These animals, he learned, were suspected of carrying FMD. Curious about the implications, Dr Packer contacted the scientists at PIADC.

They followed up on Dr Packer's tip and conducted a formal study in PIADC's secure Biosafety Level 3 facility. Their results showed that IRT photography could detect elevated hoof temperatures up to two days before cattle developed clinical signs.

"By looking at the hottest spot in the hooves, we could identify FMD infected cattle when that temperature was higher than 34.4°C," Dr Rodriguez says. "It allowed us to predict with up to 88 percent confidence which animals would develop symptoms within 48 hours."

In an IRT photograph of a group of cattle, the hooves of healthy animals appear blue-green, whereas infected cattle have orange-red feet. This easy visual distinction could allow scientists and veterinarians to identify potentially infected cattle in large groups without examining animals individually. The technology is cheaper and faster than existing screening methods, which involve individual clinical examinations for every animal.

IRT can be paired with other ARS-developed tools for superior disease-outbreak response. One such tool is a rapid diagnostic test Plum Island scientists developed in response to a 2002 request from the US Congress.

The PIADC scientists collaborated with the biotechnology company Tetracore to develop the test, which can detect RNA from the FMD virus in less than two hours. It uses technology known as 'real-time PCR'. USDA's Animal and Plant Health Inspection Service has adopted the test and uses it in the National Animal Health Laboratory Network. In the event of an FMD emergency, laboratories throughout the United States could use the test to diagnose samples rapidly. It can also be used to quickly distinguish between FMD and vesicular stomatitis, an animal disease with similar symptoms that occasionally crops up in the United States.

A Safer, Better Vaccine

Another important FMD development from PIADC is the world's first effective molecular-based FMD vaccine for cattle, developed by chemist, Marvin Grubman, and colleagues. The vaccine can be produced without using infectious FMD materials, which means it can be produced safely, in the United States, without expensive, high-containment facilities.

Another benefit is that animals vaccinated with Dr Grubman's vaccine do not produce all the antibodies that infected animals produce. Because of this, they can easily be distinguished. Most existing vaccines cause animals to produce the same antibodies as infected animals, making it difficult to determine whether an animal with antibodies was naturally infected or vaccinated.

At the ARS Plum Island Animal Disease Centre in Orient Point, New York, wildlife ecologist Craig Packer (left) and microbiologist Luis Rodriguez use an infrared thermography camera to identify cattle infected with foot and mouth disease virus.

ARS – in collaboration with the US Department of Homeland Security's Targeted Advanced Development unit and GenVec, Inc., a biopharmaceutical company based in Gaithersburg, Maryland – is developing this technology for potential commercialisation.

Tests have shown that the vaccine becomes effective a mere seven days after it has been administered. Although this is one of the fastest vaccines available, Dr Grubman and his colleagues wanted faster protection. After all, a lot can happen in seven days, particularly during an outbreak. In a recent study, Dr Grubman found that interferons – proteins produced by the immune system – can offer protection during that first week.

Interferons are so named because they interfere with virus replication. Dr Grubman and his colleagues introduced type I and type II interferon genes into an adenovirus, which they administered to groups of pigs. One day later, they infected the swine with FMD virus. The interferons blocked FMD virus replication, offering the swine protection. "The interferon gives early protection for three to five days while the animals are developing an antibody response to the vaccine," Dr Grubman says. "This significantly increases their chances of resisting FMD."

ARS and GenVec are now collaborating to combine the interferons and the FMD vaccine so they can be administered together.

Health and Welfare of Cattle Transported in Late Pregnancy

.Since July 2009 the Veterinary Laboratories Agency (VLA) has investigated the deaths of dairy heifers transported from Europe in late pregnancy. They died from severe metabolic disease within six weeks of transport, with fatty liver being the most common feature.

Further cases have included death and dehydration of pregnant heifers during transport. Metabolic disease only occurs in certain batches of heifers transported in late pregnancy, possibly associated with animals in very good or over-fat condition at calving. However, while thousands of cattle are regularly transported without apparent incident, it is recommended that pregnant cattle, and in particular heifers, should be carefully managed before, during and after long journeys.

Since 2008 Animal Health has reported a number of incidents of cattle calving during or just after transportation, contrary to current EU regulations.

There are significant risks to the health and welfare of heifers and cows transported over long distances in late pregnancy. The risk may be greater in heifers because they tend to have a shorter pregnancy and because more of them are transported when pregnant (the number of imported dairy heifers has increased in the past two years). Additionally, since most pregnant heifers are physically immature during pregnancy they may be more susceptible to the stress of long distance transport.

Farmers (both vendors and purchasers) and hauliers must be aware of these risks, take action to mitigate them, and be aware of their statutory obligations. Council Regulation EC/1/2005 lays down the provisions on the protection of animals during transport.

This is enforced in England under The Welfare of Animals (Transport) (England) Order 2006, and states that pregnant females should NOT be transported when 90 per cent or more of the expected pregnancy period has passed, or in the week after calving.

Important Factors to Consider When Transporting Pregnant Cattle

Energy and water requirements increase considerably in late pregnancy. Evidence indicates some heifers experience significant negative energy balance during transport, while others suffer from dehydration.

There may be an interruption in food and water intake (even if it is provided to the animals) during transport, particularly on long journeys.

A significant change in dietary management in late pregnancy is more likely to lead to metabolic disease. In some cases, heifers reared indoors at the source farm were put out to grass at the destination farm.

The stress of transportation may intensify these problems and lower animals' resistance to disease.

The Law on Transportation

It is an offence to transport any animal in a way which causes it, or is likely to cause it, injury or unnecessary suffering. Transporters and keepers can be prosecuted if they flout the law. In addition, animals which are unfit must not be transported. This includes pregnant dairy cattle transported in the final 10 per cent of their gestation period (with the exception of transportation for veterinary treatment), and in the week following calving.

In addition, under the Animal Welfare Act 2006, animal owners and keepers of animals have a duty of care to provide for their basic needs and to prevent suffering. Someone responsible for an animal, who permits another person to cause unnecessary suffering, is also committing an offence.

This is also the case if they fail to take reasonable steps to prevent suffering during and after transport. Intra-Community Trade Animal Health Certificates clearly state the requirements for compliance with the European Transport Regulation EC/1/2005.

Best Practice and Recommended Actions

Whilst there are legal limitations regarding the transportation of pregnant cattle in the final 10 per cent of gestation, there are increased risks to cattle health and welfare throughout pregnancy. Therefore the journey must be planned and managed to reduce these risks and to ensure that their metabolic requirements will be fully met. Check exact insemination or service date and expected calving date for each animal in the batch.

Avoid negative energy balance in late pregnancy by ensuring appropriate feeding before, during and after transport.

Avoid sudden changes of management and diet for pregnant animals. Upon arrival at the farm of destination, heifers should initially remain on the same diet as before transportation and new foods should be introduced gradually.

It is recommended that pregnant cattle are not transported over long distances in the last two months of pregnancy. This will also allow the animal to adapt to new rearing conditions before calving.

Always consider the disease status of new animals introduced in any herd. This is especially important if the animals originate from abroad because they may carry diseases that are not already present in GB. The biosecurity of the herd of destination should be managed through a herd health plan.

Cold Stress in Cows: What iCold to a Cow?

When temperatures start to decline in winter, particularly as we get closer to 0°C (or 32°F), it is time to think about what effect this is having on cow productivity and efficiency.

Like all mammals, cows are warm blooded and need to maintain a constant core body temperature. Normal rectal temperature for a cow is around 38°C (101°F).

Within a range of environmental temperatures called the "thermoneutral zone," animals do not have to expend any extra energy to maintain their body temperature.

At the lower end of this range, normal metabolic processes supply enough heat to maintain body core temperature. Within their thermoneutral zone, animals may modify their behaviour, such as seeking shelter from wind, and respond over the long term by growing a thick hair coat for winter, without affecting their nutrient requirements.

However, below the lower limit of the thermoneutral zone, in the "lower critical temperature," the animal experiences cold stress. To combat cold stress, the animal must increase its metabolic rate to supply more body heat. This increases dietary requirements, particularly for energy. Typical lower critical temperatures for beef cattle are affected by a number of factors. Table 1, below, shows the impact that different hair coat types can have on lower critical temperature.

Cattle, like humans, actually experience the "effective temperature," which takes into account both air temperature and the effect of wind chill. Cool or cold wind passing over an animal draws heat away from it much more quickly than still air at the same temperature. Wind chill effects for cattle are shown in Table 2, below. These figures assume a dry, clean hair coat. If the animal is wet and/ or dirty, consider the data to be an underestimation of the effect of the wind.

Assumes that hair coat is dry and clean.

For example, when air temperature is –18°C and wind speed is 24 kph, the effective temperature experienced by the animal is the equivalent of a still air temperature of –26°C.

If cows are exposed to wind or drafts, it is important to adjust for the effective temperature and take the appropriate steps to ensure that the cows can maintain body temperature and weight.

Factors Affecting an Animal's Ability to Withstand the Cold

- Acclimation: Cattle do adjust or acclimate to colder weather by growing a longer, thicker coat. This provides additional insulation against cold weather. The coat must be clean and dry to provide maximum protection to the cow. Dirt or moisture on the coat reduces its insulation value dramatically.
- Fat Layer: Cattle in good condition with a thick fat layer are better able to withstand the cold than thin cattle. The fat layer acts as another insulating layer between the animal's core and the environment.
- Metabolic Rate: Cows will also increase their metabolic rate to increase heat production and help maintain body temperature. This increases the need for dietary energy, so appetite is usually increased and cows eat more.

The Effects of Severe Cold Stress on Cattle

Hypothermia occurs when the body temperature drops well below normal. In general terms, with cattle, mild hypothermia occurs with a body temperature of 30°C–32°C, (86°F–89°F), moderate hypothermia at 22°F–29°C, (71°F–85°F) and severe hypothermia below 20°C (68°F). As rectal temperature drops below 28°C (82°F), cows are not able to return to normal temperature without assistance through warming and the administration of warm fluids. As hypothermia progresses, metabolic and physiological processes slow down, and blood is diverted from the extremities to protect the vital organs. Teats, ears and testes are prone to frostbite. In extremes, respiration and heart rate drop, animals lose consciousness and die.

In most situations, a more insidious and costly problem occurs. Cows are subjected to an environmental temperature below the lower critical temperature, but without obvious signs of hypothermia. This increases the maintenance energy requirement of these animals as they adjust to the conditions and divert more energy to maintaining body temperature.

There are two potential responses to this situation.

Cows have access to higher quality feed and/or increased intake, and therefore maintain their body weight.

Cows try to increase feed intake in an effort to meet their energy requirements. Given the opportunity and gut capacity, cows will eat more feed to help meet their increased energy demands. Practically, it is usually expedient to feed grain as well. This increases feed costs, increasing the cost of keeping cows, however the expectation is that cows will maintain their body weight!

It is generally accepted that for every 1°C drop below the lower critical temperature, there is an approximately 2% increase in energy requirements. The amounts of additional feed required for a cow under cold stress can be calculated, but as a rule of thumb, a cow with a dry winter coat should be fed the additional feed as presented in Table 3, below.

Cows may not be able to eat the amount of extra hay required to maintain their body weight and may have to be fed the indicated amount of grain instead of additional hay to meet their energy requirements.

Cows don't have increased feed quality and intake and lose body weight.

If cows are not fed additional feed or the quality does not allow them to eat enough to meet their additional energy requirements, body mass will be "burned" to produce metabolic heat. These cows lose weight as both feed energy and stored fat are diverted to maintain body temperature and vital functions.

Cows in this situation that start to lose weight soon enter a downward spiral — the more weight (fat) they lose, the less insulation they have, the more susceptible they are to further cold stress, and they lose weight even faster.

Cows, and especially heifers that lose weight, calve in poor condition. The consequences are increased calving difficulties, an increase in the number of lighter, weak calves and higher calf mortality. These dams produce a reduced amount of colostrum (of lower quality) and have lower milk production, increased neonatal mortality and reduced growth rate in surviving calves. These cows usually have delayed return to estrus, longer days open and poorer reproductive success.

Key management factors to limit the effects of cold stress :

- Monitor the weather. Monitor temperature and increase feeding in response to cold weather. Cows in the last trimester require additional grain feeding during periods when the effective temperature falls below the lower critical level.
- Protect animals from the wind. Wind markedly reduces the effective temperature, increasing cold stress on animals.

- Bed cows well. Providing adequate dry bedding makes a significant difference in the ability of cattle to withstand cold stress.
- Keep cows clean and dry. Wet coats have greatly reduced insulating properties and make cows more susceptible to cold stress. Mud-caked coats also reduce the insulating properties of the hair.
- Provide additional feed. Feed more hay and grain. If wet feeds are fed, make sure they are not frozen.
- Provide water. Make sure cows have ample water available at all times. Limiting water will limit feed intake and make it more difficult for cows to meet their energy requirements. Frozen troughs and excessively cold water seriously limit water intake.

We can't control the weather but we can do everything reasonably possible to reduce the effects of cold on cows. This will help reduce costs and improve production efficiency.

Nursing Calf Deworming

Carter and Matthew J. Hersom Published by the University of Florida IFAS Extension. Historically, the predominant health problem worldwide for ruminant animals has been the presence of internal parasites.

The continued use of anthelmintics, or dewormers, remains controversial among researchers because there is wide variation among results when these products are used on cattle with moderate to low levels of parasite infestation. It is clear, however, that with any level of infestation above moderate, dewormers provide almost immediate responses and improvement in animal health and performance.

Parasitic infection and disease receives relatively little attention in most areas. Likely, we are so accustomed to treating our cattle on a routine basis that clinical signs of disease are rarely observed. Immunity to parasites increases with age. Older animals like mature cows in particular have the ability to ward off many parasitic challenges, or at least keep these invaders to a minimum.

Parasites, however, may be silent rustlers of performance while existing in a sub-clinical fashion in your herd. Although these infections may not be significant enough to manifest clinical signs, weaning weights may be improved when nursing calves are dewormed at branding, or approximately three months of age. In fact, deworming calves may be the most profitable task you can perform.

If you think the effect of any given parasite stops simply with lower weight gains and an unthrifty appearance, you may be misinformed. Parasites can contribute to other conditions like anemia which can be significant because of its affect on red blood cells and thus, oxygen transport. They may also affect the immune system's ability to respond to vaccines by producing lower-than-normal white-cell populations within the body.

Beef cattle are susceptible to various parasites. Here are a few species that are important. Check with your local veterinarian for an appropriate deworming program for your herd. Be sure that you are aware of liver flukes in your area and whether or not your herd is exposed to these, as well. Not all dewormers are labelled for the control of flukes, so check your products carefully and again, consult your veterinarian.

Gastrointestinal Roundworms

- Ostertagia ostertagi
- Cooperia oncophora
- Haemonchus placei
- Trichostrongylus spp.
- Strongyloides papillosus.

Lungworms—Dictyocaulus Viviparous

Standard procedure for parasite control at most beef operations in the U.S. is to treat beef cows once or twice annually and possibly to deworm the calf at weaning only. Recent field trials have dismissed the dogma that calves did not have a sufficiently high level of parasitism to warrant treatment until weaning, or after. Industry-funded research has recently demonstrated higher weaning weights of calves treated with doramectin (Dectomax™, Pfizer Animal Health, New York) prior to weaning. Their data indicated a 25 lb advantage in weaning weight resulting in additional profit per head ($17.65), as well as a nearly four-fold return on investment (ROI) over the cost of the deworming product alone.

Deworming Calves Still on the Cow

Spring born calves (n=567) from three geographically different locations within the University of Florida/IFAS system were utilised to conduct a nursing calf deworming experiment: NFREC (MAR;

n=177), Marianna, FL; Beef Research Unit (BRU; n=186), Gainesville, FL; and Boston Farm – Santa Fe River Ranch (SF; n=204), Santa Fe, FL. At least two breed types were available at each location, including Angus, Brangus, Brahman, and Romosinuano, as well as some graded combinations of these breeds (composites).

Although processing calendar dates varied by location, the project began after June 1, 2005 and depended on the projected weaning date determined by each unit manager. Treatments included a control group (CONT), which received no deworming compounds during the study, and a treatment group (DW) which was dewormed with injectable doramectin (1 mL per 110 lb BW, subcutaneous [SC]) 90 days prior to the projected weaning date. Calves were blocked by site and randomly assigned to either CONT or DW; equal numbers were assigned to treatments as much as possible and necessary to balance the experimental design.

On day 0 all calves were individually weighed in order to get an accurate body weight which was used to calculate an appropriate dosing rate for DW. After weighing on day 0 calves were returned to their dams and taken to designated pastures for grazing. Cow-calf pairs within each unit and among treatment groups were grazed on similar forage types and received similar nutrition at all times in order to avoid bias based on forage or nutrition limitations. Treatment groups were intermingled as necessary depending on pasture conditions and overall grazing logistics. Dams were body condition scored (BCS) on day 0 of the study and at weaning to determine if any change in calf growth rate caused by the treatments may have had an indirect effect on the physical condition of the dam. Calf weights and dam BCS were also obtained at a midpoint during the study.

Pasture forage allowance was measured as cow-calf pairs were introduced to new grazing sites and when they were removed in order to estimate forage consumption during grazing.

Results

Performance data from this study are presented in Table 1 and Table 2. Across all locations, DW calves gained more total weight and ADG was greater among DW calves compared with CONT calves. On average in this experiment, deworming cost approximately $1.57 per head. DW calves returned $9.57 per head more net revenue ([lb total wt. gain x $1.28/lb BW average sale price of calves]-$1.57/hd deworming cost) when considering only the cost of the deworming product. Labour costs should be considered.

Implications

Under these experimental conditions, these data indicated both an animal performance advantage and a positive ROI. Given these results and the only modest economic improvement, economies of scale may limit the acceptance of this process to larger operations. The cost:benefit ratio may not be as significant for the average producer, especially if it means putting the herd through the chute an additional time. Labour costs, if calculated at two dollars per head, could consume nearly twenty percent of the increased revenue. Dollar value gains in the range of $15-$25 would likely make this more widely attractive. Of course this equation has various components that affect the outcome directly: calf prices, calf quality, animal performance as affected by rainfall and/or forage availability, labour and processing, etc. Some economists, however, may advise serious consideration of any procedure that adds as little as one dollar to the bottom line of any enterprise.

Ultrasound Scanning Beef Cattle for Body Composition

Ultrasound technology uses sound waves to develop images of body composition. Body composition traits that can be measured include 12th to 13th rib fat thickness, rump fat thickness, ribeye area, and intramuscular fat percentage (marbling). Each of these traits is at least moderately heritable and is significant in the determination of red meat quality and yield for individual animals.

Chapter 9

Body Composition Traits

Rib Fat

Rib fat (also called fat thickness or backfat) is an external fat measurement taken between the 12th and 13th ribs. It is measured in inches. Rib fat is used in USDA yield grade calculation and is the most important determinant of retail yield. Higher amounts of rib fat decrease cutability and produce less desirable yield grades.

Ribeye Area

Ribeye area is the surface area of the longissimus dorsi (ribeye) muscle at the 12th rib interface on the beef forequarter. Ribeye area is expressed in square inches. Retail product yield increases and numerical yield grade decreases as ribeye area increases. This image is often the most difficult to collect and requires a highly skilled interpreting technician. Both rib fat and ribeye area are taken from the same image.

Rump Fat

Rump fat refers to the depth of fat at the juncture of the gluteus medius and superficial gluteus medius muscles. This measurement is expressed in inches. It is taken from an image collected between the hooks (hips) and pins of the animal. The rump fat measurement, together with the rib fat measurement, is used to determine more accurately the overall external body fat. This improves the accuracy of predicting percent retail product. In most cases, an animal will exhibit more fat over the rump than the rib, so often more variation is displayed in rump fat measurements than rib fat measurements. This image is highly repeatable and is the least difficult to collect or interpret.

Scanning locations on the live animal are illustrated. Intramuscular fat percentage is measured at position 1, ribeye area and rib fat thickness are measured at position 2, and rump fat thickness is measured at position 3.

Intramuscular Fat

Intramuscular fat percentage (%IMF) is the percentage of fat in the ribeye muscle. It is often called marbling and is observed as flecks of fat in lean tissue. Degree of marbling is related to intramuscular fat percentage and is the primary factor determining quality grade (Table 1). Higher levels of intramuscular fat improve quality grade. This measurement should be collected when cattle are maintaining a high level of nutrition. The field technician collects four images, and the values generated by the interpreting software are averaged for an overall intramuscular fat percentage.

Acceptable Scanning Ages

Yearling bulls and heifers can be scanned at approximately 365 days of age to provide a good indication of how sibling steer and heifer mates will perform on the rail. Each breed association has established a window for age at scanning that must be complied with in order for the data to be used in the national cattle evaluation (Table 2). Consult with the respective breed association for current scanning age guidelines.

Barnsheets

Abarnsheet is a form that includes information such as herd ID, tattoo, sex, birth date, and registration number of each calf to be ultrasound scanned. Breed associations require that barnsheets be submitted with ultrasound scan images, so every animal scanned for breed association data submission must be on a barnsheet. For breeds that use ultrasound body composition data in expected progeny difference (EPD) calculations, barnsheet reporting is critical to ensure that scan results are properly reported to breed associations for EPD updates. For cattle not listed on preprinted barnsheets, the breeder must provide the necessary animal information to the ultrasound field technician for inclusion on the barnsheet at the time of scanning. This may be necessary if there are delays in data submission or registration and weaning performance paperwork processing.

Obtaining barnsheets before scanning is the responsibility of the cattle breeder, not the ultrasound field technician. To obtain a barnsheet from a breed association, a minimum amount of data must be on file with the association for the cattle to be scanned. Cattle must be registered with the association, and some breed associations require weaning weights before barnsheets will be created. Preprinted barnsheets often are distributed to breeders along with weaning performance reports. Barnsheets also may be accessed and printed by breed association members through breed associationWeb sites as part of their online accounts.

Review barnsheets before scanning to make sure all data needed to complete the sheets can be readily supplied at scanning. Barnsheets require the breeder to specify the contemporary grouping, management, and diet of the animals. A contemporary group describes cattle of similar age and sex that were managed the same and had performance data collected as a group.

Improper contemporary group reporting will cause performance results to be incorrect. Note that breed associations often require a minimum contemporary group size for ultrasound body composition scan data to be used in EPD calculations, for yearling adjustments, or for performance ratios to be computed.

Each breed association provides specific management or test type codes (abbreviations or numbers designating animal management, such as ranch test, central test, developing heifers, and feedlot) and diet codes (abbreviations or numbers describing how the animals were fed, such as specific thresholds for concentrate feed levels). Look on the barnsheets or breed association Web sites for keys to these codes and code descriptions, or contact the breed association directly for this information.

Arranging Ultrasound Scanning Services

An Ultrasound Guidelines Council-certified technician can perform ultrasound body composition scanning services for a fee. The U.S. Beef Breeds Council charged the UGC with responsibility for developing, maintaining, and governing the proficiency-testing protocol and standards for beef cattle ultrasound technician certification. The UGC coordinates proficiency testing and certification for image collection (field certification) and laboratory interpretation (lab certification). Scheduling for a UGC-certified technician to scan cattle often needs to be done well in advance of the desired scanning date. Breed associations may have additional breed-specific ultrasound guidelines and publish a list of technicians that are certified for the particular breed.

It may be advantageous for several producers in an area interested in having their bulls scanned to arrange for a technician to service multiple farms in one area in one trip. The Mississippi Beef Cattle

Improvement Association facilitates ultrasound body composition scanning of registered Mississippi cattle by accommodating ultrasound scanning sessions at centralised locations for multiple breeders at one time. This may help lower the cost of scanning for an individual farm by spreading the travel costs of the technician across several farms.

Preparing for Scanning

A grounded 110-volt electrical outlet must be provided for the field technician to use with the scanning equipment. Generators are not a desirable power source. Because cattle must be dry in the scanning regions, covered cattle holding and handling facilities may be needed in the event of precipitation. Severe weather may dictate that the scanning session be postponed until conditions become acceptable for scanning.

Be prepared to provide supplemental heat for scanning equipment and oil if the outside temperature is too cold. Covered or shaded cattle handling facilities are needed to keep animals out of direct or bright sunlight during scanning. This allows the field technician to view the images on the monitor.

Cattle should be restrained in a squeeze chute with side panel doors during scanning to ensure image quality and ease of scanning. Cattle must be adequately clipped (within one-half of an inch; many technicians clip shorter than this) and cleaned in the region of scanning. Check with the field technician in advance to decide if the breeder needs to provide clippers, electrical extension cords, vegetable oil, paper towels, or other supplies at scanning. It may be useful to keep an extra set of clippers and clipper blades on hand in the event that there is a problem with the original clippers used.

Scanning and Image Processing

Individual animal weights must be recorded within 7 days of when the cattle are scanned. Record these weights on the barnsheets for the technician to submit to the authorised image interpretation lab along with the ultrasound images. Ideally, weights are collected at the time of scanning to reduce the number of times cattle must be handled. Some breeders choose to collect all yearling performance data (weights, scrotal circumference measurements, hip heights, temperament scores) at the same time cattle are ultrasound scanned for body composition. If the scan weight is to be used as a yearling weight, the breeder must submit the weight as a yearling weight to the breed association. This weight will not automatically be used as a yearling weight.

The ultrasound field technician should submit collected images and associated completed barnsheets to an authorised lab for interpretation. Breeders must be sure to leave barnsheets with scanning technicians instead of submitting them to the breed association. The field technician should be familiar with breed association requirements regarding acceptable image interpretation labs.

Image processing fees typically are charged for image interpretation services. The ultrasound field technician may pay these fees directly and then include the charge in an invoice to the breeder or may request that the breeder send payment directly to the authorised lab. After scan data interpretation is completed, scan results are then sent to the respective breed association(s) for adjustments and EPD calculations. Breed associations then provide summaries of scanning results and related performance information to breeders.

Ask the field technician how long it generally takes for image processing to be completed and results reported to the breed association and/or breeder. Breeders will typically be notified by scanning technicians if errors are found during image processing or by breed associations during report processing. Potential errors can include bad or missing images, incomplete barnsheets, unpaid scanning or image processing fees, missing weaning weights, or animals not found in breed association databases. If an unreasonable amount of time passes after scanning with no feedback on results, contact the scanning technician and/or breed association to track down and help resolve any potential problems. Results may be reported by e-mail, mail, or member-specific screens on breed association Web sites.

Conclusions

Ultrasound scanning technology is a useful tool for collecting body composition data on live animals. The resulting data are less expensive and time consuming to collect compared with actual harvest data from beef carcasses. This technology allows seedstock producers to collect body composition data on prospective breeding animals for use in genetic improvement efforts. Ultrasound scanning results help breeders select cattle that best fit market specifications. This information provides breeders with powerful information for seedstock marketing as well.

Cattle Genetics Decoded

A powerful new selection tool can predict a calves genetic potential in our herds shortly after it's born.

The U.S. Department of Agriculture (USDA) will release genetic evaluations using genome information in January 2009, and the Canadian Dairy Network (CDN) plans to follow later in the year.

The genome of an organism, in this case a dairy animal, is its DNA-encoded hereditary information. Genome selection, coupled with already sophisticated evaluation and selection procedures, will greatly enhance efficiency and accuracy of genetic improvement programs.

Canadian and U.S. genetic improvement labs, facilities and artificial insemination (AI) studs have co-operated to develop Genomic Estimated Breeding Values (GEBVs). They are expected to revolutionize dairy breeding programs by changing the way bulls and cows are selected.

This was the message from the recent meeting of the International Committee on Animal Recording in Niagara Falls, N.Y. Highlighting the meeting were two important reports, one by Dr. George Wiggans on the co-operative effort among American and Canadian industry partners to develop genomic selection, and the other by the University of Guelph's Dr. Larry Schaeffer on how this technology can be used in an AI selection program. Together, their reports answer key questions dairy breeders are asking:

What is Genomic: Selection?

Genomic selection uses information about an individual animal's genetic make up to estimate its breeding value. Scientists developed whole genome scans using a DNA chip that identifies up to 54,000 tiny bits of genetic information. Each bit of information is called a SNP.

What are SNPs?

SNPs (pronounced snips) are like markers indicating common types of genetic variation. They can be beneficial, harmful or have no known effect.

The cattle genome has millions of SNPs. The more we find, the more we can learn about overall dairy genetics. Although not all 54,000 SNPs identified so far have proven useful in dairy genotyping, a lot of them can now help predict whether we are selecting an animal with the traits we want.

How does Selection Work?

The first step in the two-step process compares the genetic makeup of a large number of individuals with common characteristics in the general dairy cattle population. This includes milk production, calving ease, type traits and so forth.

The second step uses the information from SNPs found in each animal's genome to predict its breeding value. Computer programs add up all the effects on a given trait identified with the various SNPs. This is combined with the Parent Average used in the traditional genetic evaluation system to calculate an overall GEBV.

As Accurate as Progeny Proofs?

In the USDA project, GEBVs were estimated for 5,825 bulls and cows, and then compared with their actual 2008 breeding values to determine GEBV accuracy. This was done for production traits as well as functional, calving and type traits.

A GEBV will have a reliability factor between the Parent Average and a traditional progeny proof. The relative reliability of Parent Average is 25 to 40 per cent, depending on the trait and amount of information available on the parents. In Canada, a newly proven bull may have a proof with a reliability of 80 to 85 per cent, and proofs for bulls with large numbers of daughters will have a reliability level in the 95 per cent range.

The new GEBVs will combine genotype information from individual animals with Parent Averages, plus any individual proof information if it's available. When the USDA added genotype information plus Parent Averages, the GEBVs for bulls had a reliability ranging between 63 and 75 per cent. These reliabilities may be somewhat overestimated and may prove lower when this program is widely used.

We cannot rely on GEBVs as we would on highly proven progeny proofs, but GEBVs are much more accurate than Parent Average. With females, a GEBV is probably far more reliable than any current genetic evaluation for all but a few exceptional cows, and has the advantage of being available very early in life.

What are the Benefits?

Genomic selection has two advantages: speed and lower cost.

Genotypes can be obtained shortly after the birth of a calf that may potentially be used in AI or as a bull mother. When combined with Parent Averages to create GEBVs, the process could speed up genetic trends by 30 to 50 per cent, depending upon the accuracy of GEBVs and the extent to which the industry uses them.

A full genome scan for an individual will cost $250 to $300, compared with $40,000 to progeny-prove a single bull. This test could screen a large number of young sires to select a few to enter into progeny testing. That would potentially improve the rate of genetic gain but at a much lower cost than the current progeny testing program.

Improved reliability from GEBVs may enhance selection to improve low heritability traits such as health, fitness and fertility.

What about Inbreeding?

Since genomic selection can more accurately identify the best superior sires at a young age, it might contribute to higher rates of inbreeding. Breeding programs usually concentrate on achieving the best genetics as quickly as possible.

On the other hand, genomic selection used as a widespread screening method could identify bulls and cows of high genetic merit traditional animal model evaluations would miss.

What about Single Genes Identified as Important?

Genome-wide selection has rendered useless the approach of identifying single genes as having a positive or negative effect on an economically important trait. Multiple genes control most of these traits and act in an additive nature.

Individual genes identified as important, when included in genome-wide selection, can contribute to overall GEBV accuracy. Identifying more of these genes in years to come would likely improve reliability in the future.

Effect on AI Programs?

The advantage of GEBVs would be to pre-screen bulls before entering them into progeny testing, increasing the pace of genetic gain. However, they would still go through the same waiting period to receive a progeny-test EBV before being used in the population.

A more aggressive approach would genotype 2,000 or more young bulls but only enter a reduced number into progeny testing at one year of age. Instead of 400 bulls entering progeny testing per year, there might be only 200, and they would have been drawn from a much wider pool than they are now.

As well, a few of the best genotyped bulls would be used as sires of sons before completing their progeny tests. This method would produce 30 to 50 per cent more genetic gain than a traditional progeny test system at about the same or lower cost.

Will We Need Records Anymore?

We will still need records to identify truly superior AI sires. Progeny tests will continue since they are more reliable than GEBVs but we will probably be progeny testing much fewer bulls.

A large number of records for all economically important traits will be necessary to continue to estimate the SNP effects so we can produce more accurate GEBVs in future.

What about Cows?

A GEBV will improve the reliability of estimating the true breeding value of most cows. Typically, except for a few elite cows, we have less information to estimate true genetic merit for cows than for progeny-proven bulls. Genotyping females shortly after birth could provide relatively reliable breeding values.

AI studs interested in bull dams will probably have genotyping done on a large number of prospective females. If you have marketable females that are not the sort AI studs currently want, genotyping at less than $250 per animal could be a good option.

Emergency Considerations for Beef Cattle

The following guide is a general overview of beef cattle handling, care, and health concerns which may be associated with a natural disaster such as a hurricane.

Behaviour, Handling, Animal Care

Handling practices can be less stressful to the animals and safer for the handler if one understands the behavioural characteristics of beef cattle. Cattle disposition or temperament ranges from docile to wild/highly excitable. Typically cattle with poor dispositions are very fearful of humans or they exhibit aggressive behaviour. This behaviour is neutralised when personnel handling cattle are experienced and understand the flight zone of cattle.

Behaviour During Handling and Restraint

Cattle have a "flight zone." The flight zone of an animal is that space surrounding the animal that will elicit avoidance or escape when encroached upon. When a person moves inside the flight zone, the animal usually moves away. If a handler penetrates the flight zone too deeply (that is gets relatively close to the animal), the animal will either bolt and run, or, if cornered, turn back and run past, or over the handler.

The best place for the handler to work cattle is on the edge of the flight zone. In this position the cattle will move away from the handler in an orderly manner (will not show extreme flight behaviour). The cattle will stop moving when the handler retreats from the flight zone. The size of the flight zone of cattle depends on their relative degrees of tameness. The flight zones for cattle reared on the range may be many times greater than the flight zones of backyard or small farm cattle. It should be noted that excessively tame cattle can be very difficult to move or handle. Often the best approach is to try to get the animals to follow another animal.

The flight distance (distance from the animal to the edge of the flight zone) can be roughly estimated by walking toward the animal and noticing how close the animal may be approached before it starts to move away.

Flight distance can also be influenced by previous experience. Animals that have been handled gently and reared in close contact with people will have shorter flight distances than those that have been handled roughly or with minimal human contact.

Many people make the mistake of invading the flight zone too deeply when driving livestock. If the animals attempt to turn back, the handler should retreat from their flight zone. Retreating will usually terminate their escape behaviour.

All species of livestock exhibit a strong tendency to follow. Both sheep and cattle are highly motivated to maintain visual contact with each other. Cattle show visible signs of distress when isolated. A lone steer or cow may injure itself trying to rejoin its herd mates and if highly aroused it may also charge a handler. When a lone animal refuses to move or is agitated, either leave it alone or try to introduce it to another group of animals.

Cattle can be handled most effectively by a person who understands their behaviour patterns and who provides handling facilities that complement those behaviours in a positive way. Calm cattle are easier to move and sort than excited cattle. Once they are agitated it takes cattle about one-half hour to calm down.

Most cattle are restrained and handled several times during their lifetimes. Ease of handling depends largely on their temperament, size, and previous experience as well as on the design of the handling facilities. Cattle are also creatures of habit and will learn from positive experiences. Some cattle will move/handle easily in response to a positive motivator such as feed.

Following are some important facts about the behaviour of cattle.

1. Because cattle have 310-to 360-degree vision, they are sensitive to shadows and unusual movements.
2. Cattle tend to move toward light. (Except blinding direct sunlight.)
3. Cattle have poor depth perception and will often refuse to move through areas where shadows are cast on the ground.
4. Cows and calves handled in an abusive manner develop poor dispositions. Cattle remember painful and adverse experiences.
5. A small flag on the end of a stick is useful for moving or sorting cattle. Cattle should be moved without the use of a whip or electric prod.
6. Cattle usually respond negatively to abuse, loud noises, and other confusing situations that can excite them. Thus noisy equipment should be kept as far as possible from cattle.
7. Metal chutes and alleys should be constructed and used so as to eliminate loud clanging and banging noises.
8. Yelling at cattle increases the stress level of both cattle and handler.
9. Cattle are easily disturbed by loud noises, such as those made by pumps, and compressed air.
10. Cattle are creatures of habit. An established daily routine will result in ease of handling.
11. Handle animals in groups. A single animal will often resist going into a chute or pen by itself. It may become excited and injure itself or the handler.
12. The cattle handler's movements should be slow and deliberate: any sudden movement will frighten cattle and make them difficult to handle.
13. By understanding the flight zone of cattle, a handler can effectively work cattle in a corral or pasture.

Cattle can be moved more easily if the handler works on the edge of the flight zone.

The handler penetrates the flight zone to start cattle movement and retreats outside the flight zone to stop cattle movements. When the handler is positioned behind the point of balance at the shoulder, the animal will move forward. It will move backward when the handler is in front of the point of balance.

The animal will move forward when the handler walks quickly past the point of balance at the shoulder.

If cattle refuse to move through a gate, into a chute or trailer, or even in a certain direction, check for distractions such as flapping coats, noise, objects on the ground, other animals (dogs), movement of people in direction of travel.

Round pens enhance cattle movement and prevent injury to excitable cattle.

Head catches are necessary to immobilise cattle of large sizes. If the head needs to be restrained, a halter is preferred to nose tongs.

Mixing groups of cattle can add to the stress of these animals and make handling more difficult. If groups are mixed, provide plenty of space and observe animals from a distance. Allow the new group to interact and start to develop a social order. The anxiety will be at the highest level for the first few hours after being mixed and will decline fairly rapidly over a few days.

Breed Differences

The breed of livestock can affect the way they react to handling. Brahman and Brahman cross cattle are more excitable and may be harder to handle than the English breeds. Angus cattle may be more excitable than Herefords, and Holstein cattle tend to move slowly.

Brahman cattle often display excitement or agitation by swishing their tails. When Brahman and Brahman cross cattle become excited, they can become more difficult to block at gates, may more readily run into fences and will run over the handlers.

Brahman cattle tend to be docile in the pasture but can be claustrophobic in the pens. They are also more intelligent than English breeds. This fact results in Brahman cattle being difficult to handle when they have had previous negative experiences during handling.

Well-Being and Animal Care

Animal care aims to fulfill animal needs. In order to know how to care for animals, their needs must be known and understood.

Physiologic Needs: Nutrition, Environment or Housing, Health

Beef cattle are ruminants and are thus able to use feed stuffs such as hay and grass. If possible provide cattle with access to grass pastures. If grass pastures are not available, provide grass hay as an alternative—1/3 of a square bale/cow/day should be sufficient. Beef cattle are also able to use concentrates (grains) as a source of food. An excellent source and one which is highly palatable would be sweet feeds that are typically fed to horses. Feed approximately 10 to 12 pounds/cow/day.

In an emergency situation, mature beef cattle can survive for several days without feed.

Small calves <350 lbs nursing cows do not need additional feed, other than what is supplied to their mothers.

Orphan calves can be fed a commercial milk replacer. The amount of milk replacer supplied is typically 8% of their body weight. (i.e. a 100-lb calf would need approximately 8 lbs of reconstituted milk replacer per day). Patience is needed when trying to get an orphan calf to accept milk from a bottle or bucket, particularly if they have been used to nursing recently.

Water

Beef cattle need access to fresh water 24 hours per day. The amount of water required depends a lot upon the ambient temperature. Regardless of the types of feed supplied, beef cattle cannot go without water for any extended period of time (> 24 hours).

Beef cattle are able to use standing water as well as fresh water. Water with high levels of chlorine may be unpalatable. It has been noted by people showing cattle that animals experiencing a change in water source often decrease water consumption. Table 1 provides water requirements for cattle and other species.

Environment / Housing

A majority of beef cattle are reared in a range environment. Well-drained grass land with shade available for the entire herd should be adequate. Fencing should contain animals to a specified area. In general the smaller the area in which cattle are contained, the greater the need for higher quality fence. For example, a corral should be made of rigid material such as steel panels or wooden fencing materials or possibly woven wire. An electric fence for emergencies or a 4-5 wire permanent fence should be adequate for open pasture.

Health Concerns for Beef Cattle During an Environmental Disaster

Generally there are few if any medical emergencies for beef cattle during environmental disasters such as hurricanes.

The lack of available water may leave some animals dehydrated. The remedy is to provide fresh water as soon as possible. If an animal is severely dehydrated, fluids can be provided via a stomach tube. Adequate restraint would be necessary as well as advanced training on the technique for "tubing" a ruminant.

Lack of shade may cause heat stress or heat stroke. Moving animals during periods of high temperature and humidity may also lead animals into heat stress or stroke. Often for beef cattle in hot and humid conditions *the best thing to do to prevent heat stress is to simply leave them alone.*

Use the temperature humidity index as a guide to heat stress. Listen to local or regional weather reports for the temperature humidity index (THI) for your area.

Some levels of concern include:

- Above 75 THI-Heat stress on high-producing cows begins to decrease feed intake and lower milk production, especially in diary cows.
- Above 80 THI-Severe heat stress may occur for cows on pasture. Shade and adequate ventilation are essential to minimise stress and animal loss.
- Above 83-85 THI-Danger of fatal heat stress occurs.

Heat stress management plan should incorporate the following:

a. Have ample water available. 2-3 gallons of water per 100 lbs of body weight. Make sure of delivery capability.
b. If watering from a trough, 3 inches of linear space per animal may be lifesaving.
c. Avoid handling of cattle if at all possible.
d. Provide shade if possible.
e. Improve air flow if possible. Provide fans or ventilation for confined cattle.

Don't house animals in a small pen in direct sunlight without adequate shade, water and ventilation (air flow).

Emergency Medical Treatment

If beef cattle are in need of medical treatment during a hurricane, consider the use of local resources: local veterinarians, cowboys, and area ranchers.

If veterinary assistance is required to manage health concerns, more than likely restraint facilities will also be necessary. This will include equipment such as squeeze chutes, corrals, lariats, rope halters and possibly sedatives and or anesthetics. If facilities are needed, adequate preparation should be made accordingly. It may be necessary to consider euthanasia rather than treatment of some animals. If euthanasia is a consideration for severely injured animals, adequately trained personnel will be necessary.

Health concerns regarding debilitated, disabled, or injured cattle will often require a decision of either treatment, or euthanasia. Criteria to be considered to assist the decision making should include,

a. Pain and distress of the animal
b. Likelihood of recovery
c. Ability to get to feed and water
d. Diagnostic information
e. Welfare for the animal and humane considerations.

During an environmental disaster, beef cattle may have emergency needs for food, water, shelter and medical concerns. In reality, often the best option concerning the needs of beef cattle in a disaster, provided they are in no danger, is to note their location and the approximate number of animals, determine their ownership and then simply monitor the cattle for other needs. The owners of beef cattle, ranchers and cowhands are often the individuals best prepared to handle the emergency needs for their herds.

These individuals may need assistance from other producers in the area and occasionally local disaster relief personnel. If producers do need assistance from disaster relief personnel, volunteers providing that assistance must have a basic understanding of beef cattle. In closing, the best approach with beef cattle may be to leave the animals alone, notify local authorities if necessary, let the ranchers and cowboys handle their cattle and provide emergency assistance when producers ask for it.

Reducing Lameness in Dairy Cows

According to researchers participating in Welfare Quality®, farmers significantly underestimate the amount of lameness in their herds and in doing so, not only risk reducing the welfare of their animals but also losing some of their profits at the same time. Though farmers estimate about 5% to 10% of their dairy cows suffer from lameness, the average is closer to 25% of the herd. Lameness reduces the efficiency of a cow's milk production, with an estimated average loss of €200 per cow, per year. In other words, this welfare problem accounts for a loss of 5% to 10% of a farmer's annual income per cow.

However, thanks to research done in Welfare Quality®, some practical support has been developed that will help farmers shrink their financial losses while improving the quality of life for their cows.

A Few Practical Tips

When aiming to reduce lameness in the dairy herd, one of the first places to look is the housing system. Even in the narrow range of around one cubicle per cow, i.e. on average 0.85 to 1.15 cubicles per cow, the more cubicles there are available to a cow, the better off she will be. But not just any cubicle will do. The size of the cow in relation to the size of the cubicle is vital as are the softness and cleanliness of the lying area. If the cubicle isn't up to standard, this will increase the time that it takes a cow to lie down, which is a sign the stall isn't comfortable for her.

Just as important as the cubicle is the cow's diet. As a ruminant, the amount of forage she consumes is vital to the workings of the gut, yet at the same time she requires a lot of energy to produce the amount of milk required of her. A balance must be struck so that she gets enough energy but is also given enough forage to counteract the amount of acid that can build up in her rumen and cause lameness issues.

According to research done by Welfare Quality® on herds that were fed on average 0 kg up to 0.44 kg concentrates per kg milk, the risk of lameness increases with increasing amounts of concentrates fed. However, simply reducing the amount of concentrates compromises the energy status in high producing cows so the challenge is in balancing forage and energy.

The most obvious place to look in terms of lameness is at the health of the hoof itself. Though diet can have effects on the hoof and hoof wall, it is important to keep the area where she walks and milks dry and clean from slurry. Welfare Quality® researchers looked into the best type of flooring and the answer isn't as simple as farmers might wish: cement floors, especially when slatted, new and abrasive, can damage the hoof and weaken the soles, causing lesions and eventually infections and abscesses. Also, such floors become slippery due to wear, yet alternative rubber floors are difficult to clean with standard manure scrapers and, especially when solid, can be slippery despite the soft surface. Finding a combination of favourable features of the two types of floor that works best in each particular situation may be a process of trial and error.

Getting a Handle on Monitoring

To reduce lameness in the dairy herd, it's vital for farmers to develop a monitoring and control strategy that will look at the basic steps:

- Diagnosis – what is the problem and how big is it?;
- Risk assessment – what is causing the problem?;
- Control strategies – what can be done about it?;
- And Monitoring – is progress being made?

Welfare Quality® is developing a DVD and web-based monitoring programme to assist dairy farmers in all of these steps. The programme includes worksheets that can be tailored to suit individual farms. It will be made available in English for free, welfarequality.net and we expect to advertise this service in autumn 2008 on the Welfare Quality®.

Animal welfare can be a difficult concept to pin down, and many people have their own personal views. Despite this, there is general agreement within the scientific community that animals should be housed in comfortable surroundings and maintained in good health, as described in the Welfare Quality® fact sheet 'Principles and criteria of good animal welfare'.

The research on lameness done in Welfare Quality® has added scientific knowledge about root causes. Existing and new information has been applied in a web based monitoring programme, which assists dairy farmers in addressing risk factors in a way that is tailored to their specific situation. Welfare Quality® is providing a means to effectively combat lameness in dairy cows and contribute to an economically efficient and animal friendly dairy industry.

Finding the Early Stages of Foot and Mouth Disease

The research, The Early Pathogenesis of Foot-and-Mouth Disease in Cattle After Aerosol Inoculation-Identification of the Nasopharynx as the Primary Site of Infection, which is published in the November edition of Veterinary Pathology could lead to the development of new vaccines to control and potentially eradicate FMD.

The research was carried out by J. Arzt1, J. M. Pacheco1 and L. L. Rodriguez from the Agricultural Research Service (ARS) Foreign Animal Disease Research Unit at the Plum Island Animal Disease Centre at Orient Point, New York.

The researchers said that in order to characterise the early events of foot-and-mouth disease virus (FMDV) infection in cattle following a simulated natural exposure, 16 steers were aerosol inoculated with FMDV and then killed at various times.

Serum, nasal swabs, and oral swabs samples were collected from each steer antemortem and postmortem. In all a total of up to 40 tissue samples were taken from each animal.

These were screened for FMDV by virus isolation and for FMDV RNA by real-time reverse transcription polymerase chain reaction.

Tissues that tested positive for FMDV or viral RNA were examined by immunohistochemistry and multichannel immunofluorescence microscopy.

The scientists said that in previremic steers, FMDV was most consistently discovered in the nasopharyngeal tissues, thereby indicating this region as the most important site of primary viral replication. They said that the earliest site of microscopic localisation of FMDV antigens was the lymphoid follicle-associated epithelium of the pharyngeal mucosa-associated lymphoid tissue of the nasopharynx at six hours after the aerosol inoculation.

At early time points after aerosol inoculation, viral antigens were found together with cytokeratin-positive pharyngeal epithelial cells. Intraepithelial FMDV-negative, MHCII/CD11c-double-positive dendritic cells were present in close proximity to FMDV-positive cells, the researchers said.

The onset of viremia coincided with marked increase of viral loads in pulmonary tissues and with substantial decrease of viral detection in nasopharyngeal tissues.

The research team said that the data indicate that following aerogenous exposure to FMDV, the temporally defined critical pathogenesis events involve:

1. primary replication in epithelial cells of the pharyngeal mucosa-associated lymphoid tissue crypts and
2. subsequent widespread replication in pneumocytes in the lungs, which coincides with
3. the establishment of sustained viremia.

Beef Cattle Nutritional Disorders

The National Animal Health Monitoring System reports that 7 per cent of beef cattle death losses in the southeast U.S. in 2005 were caused by digestive problems such as bloat and acidosis. Death losses from digestive problems increased as herd size decreased.

Mineral imbalances, sudden shifts from high roughage to high concentrate diets, and swallowing foreign objects are some of the factors associated with nutritional disorders in beef cattle.

Conditions associated with mineral imbalances include grass tetany, water belly, polioencephalomalacia, white muscle disease, and milk fever. Mississippi State University Extension Service Publication 2484, Mineral and Vitamin Nutrition for Beef Cattle, discusses these conditions in detail. Nutritional disorders outlined in this publication include bloat, acidosis, and hardware disease.

Bloat

Cause

Bloat is a common digestive disorder in beef cattle. It occurs most often in feedlot cattle but affects cattle in all production phases. It results when cattle can not belch (eructate) or release gases produced normally from microbial fermentation in the rumen. The animal may produce more gas than it can eliminate. Rumen expansion from gases puts pressure on the diaphragm and lungs. This compression reduces or cuts off the animal's oxygen supply and can suffocate cattle.

Frothy bloat (feedlot bloat) is the most common type of bloat. It results from foam in the rumen that stops the animal from expelling rumen gases. The foam can cover the cardia (esophageal entrance from the reticulorumen) and prevent the animal from belching. Frothy bloat occurs in cattle fed high-grain diets but is not a major concern for many Mississippi cattle producers. "Feedlot" bloat is a concern, though, with cattle on high-grain diets, such as bulls on feed-based bull development programs.

Consuming forages with high levels of soluble protein (such as alfalfa, winter wheat, and white clover) contributes to stable foam production. This is called frothy pasture bloat or legume bloat. Legumes that contain leaf tannins help break up the foam in the rumen and are rarely associated with bloat.

These tannincontaining legumes include arrow leaf clover, berseem clover, birdsfoot trefoil, sericea lespedeza, annual lespedeza, and crownvetch. Tropical legumes such as kudzu, cowpea, perennial peanut, and alyceclover rarely cause bloat. Bloat can also occur on lush annual ryegrass or small grain pastures, particularly in spring.

Free-gas bloat is another type of bloat that happens when the cardia or esophagus is obstructed or damaged or when rumen movement is depressed.

Bull displaying a distended upper left side, indicating bloat.

Clinical Signs

Cattle suffering from bloat swell rapidly on the left side and may die within an hour. Sudden death from bloat is frequently cited in feedlots as a cause of cattle losses. Cattle may show signs of discomfort by kicking at their sides or stomping their feet. Susceptibility to bloat varies with individual animals. Some animals tend to bloat when others do not.

Management Guidelines

Do not turn shrunk or hungry cattle out onto lush legume or small grain pastures without first filling them up on hay. Bloat is still possible on these forages, even after a frost. Bloat risk is lower when legumes begin to flower than with earlier plant growth. Use of forages containing condensed tannins can help prevent bloat. Slowly adapt cattle from forage-based diets to grain-based diets over a period of at least three weeks. Manage the nutritional programs of chronic bloaters carefully.

Provide poloxalene in a salt-molasses block or as a top dressing to feed according to label recommendations. If providing poloxalene blocks, make sure cattle consume the blocks at least three days before placing the cattle on a pasture with a significant bloat risk. Remove other sources of salt, and place poloxalene blocks (30 pounds per four to five animals) where they will be easily accessible to the cattle. Feeding monensin can reduce the risk of both feedlot and pasture bloat. Monensin is reported to be more effective than lasalocid in controlling bloat, while poloxalene is more effective than monensin for bloat prevention.

Discuss bloat treatment options with a veterinarian. A veterinarian or experienced person can administer poloxalene through a stomach tube to help break up the stable foam and let the animal belch. Do not drench a bloated animal because of the danger of inhalation and then possible pneumonia or death. Feed coarsely chopped roughage as 10 to 15 per cent of the ration in a finishing diet. A bloat needle (6 to 7 inches long) or a trocar can be used in extreme cases to puncture the rumen wall on the left side of the animal to relieve pressure inside the rumen. Consider this as a last resort, because severe infections may result. Although there is no label claim, research indicates that monensin reduces the incidence and severity of frothy bloat.

Acidosis, Rumenitis, and Liver Abscesses

Cause

Acidosis is often associated with a shift from a forage based diet to a high concentrate-based diet or excessive consumption of fermentable carbohydrates. Acidosis may occur in cattle on high-grain diets common with youth livestock projects, bull development programs, and cattle finishing programs. It can also occur in stocker calves when self-feeders and highstarch feeds such as corn are used.

Acidosis is the result of low rumen pH. The typical pH of the rumen on a forage-based diet is 6 to 7. As the amount of forage or roughage in the diet decreases and the amount of concentrate increases, the pH of the rumen falls between 5 and 6, depending on the forage to concentrate ratio of the diet. Low pH supports growth of lactic acid-producing bacteria. Lactic acid is very strong and reduces rumen pH even more. Acute (severe) acidosis occurs when ruminal pH drops below 5.2, while subacute (less severe) acidosis occurs at a ruminal pH of less than 5.6. Laminitis, liver abscesses, and polioencephalomalacia often accompany acidosis.

Clinical Signs

Effects of acidosis on cattle may include slowing or stopping of gut movement (rumen stasis), diarrhea, and dehydration. Cattle appear weak, anorexic, and uncoordinated. Manure is often soft, gray, and foamy. Nutrient absorption may be impeded after animals recover from a bout of acidosis. Cattle with subacute acidosis may exhibit reduced but variable feed intake and decreased performance. Susceptibility to subacute acidosis may vary among animals. Acute acidosis can result in heart and lung failure and death.

Both subacute and acute acidosis can lead to rumenitis (infection of the rumen wall). The low pH from acidosis creates lesions in the rumen wall. Damage to the rumen wall from sharp objects (such as wire or nails) predisposes the animal to abscess formation. When rumenitis develops, liver abscesses often follow. Bacteria (*F. necrophorum, Actinomyces pyogenes, Bacteriodes spp.*) from the rumen that cause liver abscesses enter the blood supply through ulcerative lesions, hairs, or foreign objects embedded in the rumen wall. These bacteria then travel via blood to the liver.

Liver abscesses are most often seen in feedlot cattle. Severe liver abscesses may reduce feed intake, weight gain, feed efficiency, and carcass yield. Abscessed livers are condemned at harvest, regardless of abscess severity. Liver condemnations from abscesses were observed in 13.5 per cent of fed cattle in the 2005 National Beef Quality Audit, resulting in about a 2 per cent reduction in carcass weight per head. Abscesses were the primary cause of liver condemnations.

Management Guidelines

When cattle are exposed to a high-concentrate diet too quickly, acidosis may result. Fluctuations in eating behaviour are often observed. To reduce the incidence of acidosis, use a warm-up feeding period, introducing high-concentrate feeds gradually over three to four weeks. Keep at least 10 per cent roughage in the final diet to help moderate rumen pH. Forages and cottonseed hulls are both good roughage sources high in effective fibre.

While acidosis most often occurs during adaptation to concentrate-rich diets, chronic acidosis may continue into the feeding period. Feeding a combination of grains or feeding a dry grain with a high-moisture grain can reduce the risk of acidosis. Potential for acidosis is higher when feeding wheat than corn.

Processing grains less thoroughly and limiting the quantity of feed offered should reduce acidosis incidence but may also lower animal performance. Good bunk management where all feed is consumed before the next feeding may lessen daily fluctuations in feed intake and reduce acidosis risk.

Feeding ionophores (monensin or lasalocid) can help reduce the incidence of acidosis. Ionophores may reduce intake and help moderate concentrate intake when calves start on higher concentrate diets. Adding bicarbonate, fat up to 8 per cent of the diet, probiotics, virginiamycin, or thiamin to the diet or increasing protein in the diet may decrease acidosis risk.

Treatment for acidosis is similar to prevention efforts. Tylosin is effective in decreasing liver abscess incidence. Virginiamycin and chlorotetracycline also are used in addressing liver abscess problems.

Hardware Disease

Cause

Hardware disease is the common name for traumatic gastritis and traumatic reticulitis. It may occur when cattle consume sharp, heavy objects, such as nails or wire. These objects fall to the rumen floor and are swept into the reticulm by muscle contractions.

Cattle may ingest these objects and never have hardware disease, or muscle contractions may cause these sharp objects to puncture the reticulum wall, diaphragm, and heart sac. Forceful abdominal movement during calving may force a sharp object through the reticulum wall. This leads to severe damage to and infection of the abdominal cavity, heart sac, or lungs.

Clinical Signs

Signs of hardware disease vary, depending on where the puncture occurs. Loss of appetite, depression, reluctance to move, arched back, and indications of pain are common signs. The animal may grunt when forced to walk. Recurring bloat may be noticed on the upper left side, with fluid accumulation on the lower right. If the heart sac has been punctured, fluid may accumulate around the heart and in the brisket. Fatal infection can occur if the object penetrates close to the heart.

Conclusions

Knowledgeable beef cattle producers can reduce or eliminate risk factors for bloat, acidosis, and hardware disease. Watch cattle for signs of nutritional disorders to facilitate early intervention and treatment. Solicit veterinary assistance when developing and implementing treatment programs for suspect cases of nutritional disorders.

Vasoconstriction & Heat Stress Caused By Ergot Alkaloids & Fescue Toxins

Ergot alkaloids (also named ergolines) exert toxic effects in all animal species, and the most prominent toxic signs can be attributed to the interaction of ergot alkaloids with adrenergic, serotinergic and dopaminergic receptors.

Information on the chemical and toxicological properties of individual ergot alkaloids is too limited at the present time for their selection as individual marker toxins when it comes to monitoring the extent of contamination. This means that neither the total alkaloid content, nor a single alkaloid can be recommended as reliable indicators of the potential adverse effects to livestock associated with the ingestion of ergot contaminated feeds. Alkaloids have different and dose-dependent receptor selectivity (binding affinity). Consequently, the biological effects of the various complex mixtures to which animals are exposed to, remain unpredictable.

The term ergot alkaloid refers to a diverse group of about forty different toxins which are formed by Claviceps spp. on grains, triticale, corn, wheat, barley, oats, millet, sorghum and rice) and by fungal endophytes such as Neotyphodium spp. in grasses, particularly tall fescue and perennial ryegrass, which adversely affects the health and productivity of livestock. This fungus produces the ergot responsible for the ergot alkaloid group of mycotoxins and parasitizes the seed heads of plants at the time of flowering.

The main groups of natural ergot alkaloids are:

- The clavines – e.g. agroclavine
- The lysergic acids
- The lysergic acid amides – e.g. ergonovine (ergometrine, ergobasine), ergine
- The ergopeptines – e.g. ergovaline, ergotamine, ergocornine, ergocristine, ergosine, ergocryptine

The ingestion of contaminated feedstuffs by the animals can have several sources ranging from contaminated farm equipment to contaminated seed line and feeding contaminated hay or silage. Therefore, good agricultural practices that limit contamination along with feeding compounds that have the capacity to bind these toxins are needed to reduce or eliminate the harmful effects. These selected substances bind ergot alkaloids in the gastrointestinal tract, reduce their bioavailability and increase their excretion as an adsorbent-toxin complex, thus helping control the negative impacts of these mycotoxins.

Ingestion of endophyte toxins in grasses, even at sub-clinical amounts is of concern in animal production. Perennial ryegrass endophytes (Neotyphodium lolii) together with the neurotoxin lolitrem B and the vasoconstrictor ergovaline are responsible for, among others, hypersensitivity in ruminants, impaired heat stress recognition, and vasoconstriction. Plant toxins are chemical defence of plants against herbivores. Endophytic toxins in grasses include ergot alkaloids in tall fescue and tremorgens (e.g., lolitrem B) in perennial ryegrass. Perennial ryegrass endophyte (Neotyphodium lolii) alkaloids are frequently present in pastures containing the neurotoxin lolitrem B, together with the vaso-constrictor ergovaline, at levels associated with ryegrass staggers, heat stress, ill-thrift and lowered milk production. It has been shown that some of the physiological processes such as fertility may be lowered following ingestion of alkaloids produced by Neotyphodium endophytes.

Toxicity

Animals can be exposed to complex mixtures of ergot alkaloids in many typical animal agriculture production systems. This exposure results from the fact that the kinds of alkaloids present and their levels can vary widely, depending on the fungal strain, the host plant and environmental conditions, being impossible to relate the exposure to individual toxins. The chemically diverse group of ergot alkaloids has been shown in vasoconstriction symptoms, being responsible for heat intolerance as well as necrosis of ears, tails and often hooves. Other symptoms such gangrenous changes, neurotoxic signs including convulsions, abortions and death, reduced prolactin secretion and consequently agalactia have been reported as major adverse effects in animals.

Due to the fact that animals are exposed to a multiplicity of alkaloids when consuming endophyte-infected tall fescue, a combined alkaloid effect has been suggested by Klotz et al. (2008). Chronic exposure to moderate amounts of ergot alkaloids results in reduced weight gain, low reproductive efficiency, including decreased conception rates, decreased circulating progesterone, and reduced signs of estrus.

Experiments conducted in New Zealand indicate that cattle are slightly less susceptible to ergovaline toxicity than sheep with respect to live weight gain suppression. Threshold levels of ergovaline and lolitrem B have been established for cattle, sheep and horses (Table 3). These levels, however, refer to the level of toxin in the total diet, not in single feed components.

High-Density SNP Genotypes for Predicting Genetic Merit of Beef Cattle

The genetic merit of beef cattle, reported as Expected Progeny Differences (EPD), are predicted from pedigree and performance records. The fact that chromosomes are paired, and one member of each pair is transmitted from parent to offspring, results in the expected merit of offspring being the average of the parents. However, recombination between homologous chromosomes and chance sampling of chromosomes at meiosis results in some offspring that are much better than parent average and others that are much worse. Identifying the outstanding individuals is not possible until they have produced their own performance records, or better still, generated a number of performance-recorded offspring. Accurate assessment of merit is therefore not possible until well beyond puberty, the ideal selection age to provide for rapid turnover of generations.

The ability to genotype cattle for 50,000 SNP markers for around $300 has made it possible to evaluate the genetic merit of thousands of chromosome fragments identified using the markers. Given an EPD for each chromosome fragment, an animal can readily be evaluated directly from knowledge of its SNP genotypes, even in the absence of information as to its parentage. The animal's EPD is simply the sum of the EPDs of the chromosome fragments.

Coccidiosis in Beef Cattle :What is Coccidiosis?

The disease is caused by microscopic protozoan organisms known as coccidia that inhabit the cells of the intestinal lining. Each class of livestock has a species-specific coccidia; there is no cross-infection between species.

At least nine species of Bovine coccidia occur in Alberta, but only two species, Eimeria zuernii and Eimeria bovis cause the disease coccidiosis. Eggs are produced within cattle, which pass out in manure. Under proper temperatures, moisture and oxygen, sporozoites form within the egg after 3 to 7 days. These eggs then re-enter cattle if they are eaten. Sporozoites enter the intestinal cells and begin to divide, causing the cell to rupture. This allows for the spread of infection to other intestinal cells, possibly destroying many intestinal cells. After approximately 14-6 days, fertilized eggs are again produced, and pass out through manure of infected animals.

What are the Symptoms of Coccidiosis?

The severity of disease depends on several factors, including the number of eggs eaten, the species of coccidia present, and the age and condition of the animal. The symptoms usually include diarrhea varying in severity from watery manure to containing blood. Dehydration, weight loss, depression, loss of appetite and occasionally death may also occur. Even less severe infection, where there are no signs of the disease, may affect the growth and health of an animal. Additionally, nervous coccidiosis can develop in some calves with acute intestinal coccidiosis. This is usually observed in feedlot operations, especially during cold spells, with symptoms that vary in severity from minor muscular incoordination and loss of balance to intermittent or continuous seizures.

How am I sure it is Coccidiosis?

These symptoms are not specific to coccidiosis, and a veterinarian should be consulted if the above symptoms are observed. Diagnosis is made from a combination of herd history, clinical signs, physical examination of the animal and microscopic examination of manure from the rectum of the affected animal.

How does an Animal become Infected?

Bovine coccidiosis is most frequently seen in calves that are 6 to 12 months of age. Animals become infected when placed on pastures or in lots that have been contaminated by mature cattle or other infected calves. Mature cattle can also be infected when they are brought in from pastures and crowded into feedlots or barns. Most cases of coccidiosis occur during the winter months, but infection can develop whenever cattle are crowded together.

Cattle with light infections or animals that recover from coccidiosis (and usually become immune to later infections) can still continue to pass eggs in manure, and provide sources of infection for susceptible animals.

How can Infection be Prevented?

Young susceptible animals should be kept as clean and dry as possible. Feeding and watering equipment should be cleaned and protected from fecal contamination. Avoid feeding cattle on the ground, especially calves, so manure does not contaminate the feed. Excessive moisture in pens should be drained, and dry bedding should be provided.

Use pasture that are well drained, and avoid forcing animals to graze down to the roots of the plants so they do not eat large numbers of parasites. Try to keep grazing to a minimum in areas where cattle congregate (e.g. by water).

Whenever possible, infected animals should be isolated as soon as possible to avoid exposure of infected manure to other cattle.

Can Coccidiosis be Treated?

A veterinarian should always be consulted when deciding on treatment protocol. There are several anticoccidial drugs available. Outbreaks of coccidiosis in calves and feeder cattle can also be handled by mass medication using sulfonamides, amprolium or monensin added to either feed or water. Specific recommendations should be obtained from a veterinarian.

Bibliography

Alexander, D.: *Poultry Diseases,* Elsevier, 2007.

Allister, Mark Christopher: *Eco-man: New Perspectives on Masculinity and Nature,* University of Virginia Press, Charlottesville, 2004.

Archana Satarkar: *Food Science and Nutrition*, ABD Pub, Delhi, 2008.

Arora, N. : *Manual of Animal Nutrition*, International Book, 2004.

Aruna T. Kumar : *Handbook of Animal Husbandry*, Indian Council of Agricultural Research, 2008.

Balch M.D., J. and Balch C.N.C, P. : *Prescription for Nutritional Healing,* New York, U.S.A: Avery Publishing Group, 1997.

Baldick, Julian: *Animals and Shaman: Ancient Religions of Central Asia*, New York University Press, New York, 2000.

Balram Pani: *Textbook of Animal Chemistry*, I K International, Delhi, 2007.

Basu, T.K. : *About Mothers, Children, and Their Nutrition,* London, England: Thorsons Publishing, 1981.

Baudrillard: *The Animals: Territory and Metamorphoses. Simulacra and Simulation.* Ann Arbor: University of Michigan Press, 1994.

Benton, Ted: *Natural Relations: Ecology, Animal Rights and Social Justice*, Verso, London, 1993.

Betteridge, K.J. : *Embryo Transfer in Farm Animals,* Ottawa, Agriculture Canada, 1977.

Bhosale, Dinesh T. : *Handbook of Poultry Nutrition*, International Book, 2004.

Brock, J. : *A Natural History of Domesticated Animals*, Cambridge Univ. Pr., New York, 1999.

Brown, R. E.: *Social Odours in Animals Reproduction*, Clarendon Press, Oxford, 1985.

Budiansky, S.: *The Covenant of the Wild: Why Animals Chose Domestication*, Morrow, New York, 1992.

Chandra, Rajesh : *Diseases of Poultry and Their Control*, IBDCO, Delhi, 2001.

Clark, S. and S. Lyster: *Animals and Their Moral Standing,* Routledge, London, 1997.

Clark, Stephen: *The Moral Status of Animals*. Oxford: Oxford University Press, 1977.

Clymer, R. : *Nature's Healing Agents*, PA, U.S.A: Dorrance Co., 1963.

Coren, Stanley: *The Pawprints of History: Dogs and the Course of Human Events*, Free Press, New York, 2002.

Cox, N. A. : *Relationship Between Aerobic Bacteria, Salmonella, And Campylobacter on Broiler Carcasses*, Journal of Food Protection, 1997.

Crawford A. : *Experiments and Observations on Animal Heat*, London: Printed for J. Johnson; 1788.

DeGrazia, David: *Taking Animals Seriously: Mental Life and Moral Status*, Cambridge, New York, 1996.

Devender Pratap Singh : *A Handbook of Beekeeping*, Agrobios, 2006.

Dolins, Francine: *Attitudes to Animals: Views on Animal Welfare*, Cambridge University Press, Cambridge, 1999.

Donna Hill : *Biosecurity in the Poultry Industry*, International Book, 2006.

Edwards, L. : *Baking for Health*, New York, U.S.A: Avery Publishing Group, 1988.

Erasmus, U. : *Fats and Oils*, Vancouver: Alive Press, 1987.

Fairey, D.T., & Hampton, J.G. : *Forage Seed Production of Temperate Species*, Farnham Royal: CAB. 1997.

Flowerdew, J. R. : *Animals: Their Reproductive Biology and Population Ecology*, Cambridge Univ. Pr., New York, 1987.

Fox, Michael Allen: *The Case for Animal Experimentation*, University of California Press, Berkeley, CA, 1986.

Fraser, AF & Broom, DM.: *Farm Animal Behaviour and Welfare*, CABI, UK, 2004.

Gates, P.: *Animal Communication*, Cambridge University Press, Cambridge, 1997.

Guenter, W.: *Egg Nutrition and Biotechnology*, CABI Publishing, NY, 2000.

Hambidge, Gove : *Diseases and Parasites of Poultry*, Biotech Books, Delhi, 2004.

Harrison, R. J.: *Functional Anatomy of Marine Animals*, New York: Academic Press, 1974.

Homer O. Stuart: *Commercial Poultry Farming*, Biotech Books, Delhi, 2011.

Jacobson, M. : *Safe Food: Eating Wisely in a Risky World*, Washington, DC: Living Planet Press, 1991.

Katz, Jon: *The New Work of Dogs: Tending to Life, Love, and Family*, Villard, New York, 2003.

Keith Wilson N.D.P: *A Handbook of Poultry Practice*, Agrobios, Delhi, 2000.

Leclercq, B.: *Nutrition and Feeding of Poultry*, Nottingham University Press, U.K., 1994.

Mandal, A.B. : *Nutrition and Disease Management of Poultry*, International Book Distributing Co, Delhi, 2004.

Manning, Aubrey, and James Serpell: *Animals and Human Society,* Routledge, New York, 1994.

Mathialagan, P : *Textbook of Animal Husbandry and Livestock Extension,* International Book Distributing Co, Delhi, 2005.

McCollum EV. : *A history of nutrition*, Boston: Houghton Mifflin; 1957.

Moguilevsky, M. A. : *Drug Resistance of Enterobacteriacaea Isolated from Chicken Carcasses*, Journal of Food Protection, 1997.

Mohiuddin, S M : *Moulds and Mycotoxins in Poultry Diseases*, International Book, Delhi, 2007.

Morton, Eugene S.: *Animal Talk: Science and the Voices of Nature,* Random House, New York, 1992.

Nyholt, D.H. : *The Vitamin & Herb Guide,* Alberta, Canada: Global Health Ltd., 1992.

Owen, W Powell : *Poultry Farming and Keeping*, Biotech Books, Delhi, 2005.

Powell., C. : *Microbiological and Hydraulic Evaluation of Immersion Chilling for Poultry*, Journal of Food Protection, 1995.

Rakesh Kumar Shukla : *Handbook of Poultry Diseases : A Bedside-Guide*, International Book Dist, Delhi, 2006.

Randall, C.J.: *Color Atlas of Diseases and Disorders of the Domestic Fowl and Turkey,* Iowa State University Press, UK, 1991.

Raymond, F., Redman, P., & Waltham, R. : *Forage conservation and Feeding.* Ipswich: Farming Press, 1986.

Renaville, R and A Burny : *Biotechnology in Animal Husbandry*, Springer Pub, 2008.

Rifkin, Jeremy: *Beyond Beef: The Rise and Fall of the Cattle Culture*, Dutton, New York, 1992.

Rogers, Katherine: *The Cat and the Human Imagination,* The University of Michigan Press, Ann Arbor, 2001.

Sainsbury, D.: *Poultry Health and Management,* Blackwell Science, US, 2000.

Saxena, H.C. : *Poultry Feed Technology : Feed Formulation and Manufacturing*, International Book, Delhi, 2006.

Sharpe, Robert: *Science on Trial: The Human Cost of Animal Experiments*, Awareness Books, Sheffield, UK, 1994.

Short, R. V.: *Reproduction in Mammals*, Cambridge, Cambridge University Press, 1972.

Shukla, Rakesh Kumar : *Handbook of Animal Diseases : A Bedside-Guide*, International Book Dist, Delhi, 2006.

Singh, Ram Prakash : *Modern Livestock and Poultry Production*, Biotech Books, Delhi, 2008.

Snaydon, R.W. : *Managed Grasslands,* Amsterdam & London: Elsevier, 1987.

Tabor, Roger K.: *The Wild Life of the Domestic Cat,* Arrow Books, London, 1983.

Thornhill, Nancy W.: *The Natural History of Inbreeding and Outbreeding*, Chicago Press, 1993.

Thyagarajan, D. : *Diseases of Poultry*, Satish Serial pub, Delhi, 2011.

Ucko, Peter J. and G.W. Dimbleby: *The Domestication and Exploitation of Plants and Animals*, Aldine Publishing Company, Chicago, IL, 1969.

Watson, R.: *Eggs and Health Promotion,* Iowa State Press, UK, 2002.

Index

○○○